The

Paramedic

Survival

Handbook

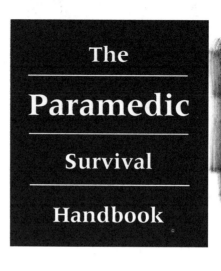

Scott W. Martin B.S., R.E.M.T.-P.
Akron General Medical Center
Akron, Ohio

A Skidmore-Roth Publication

D1522837

Printed in the United States of America

Developmental Editor: Rae Robertson
Copy Editor: Kathryn Head
Typesetting: Barbara Barr, Visual Identity
Cover Design: Barbara Barr, Visual Identity

Notice: The author and publisher of this volume have taken care to make certain that all information is correct and compatible with standards generally accepted at the time of publication. Because the field is continually changing and expanding, new techniques and concepts are continually implemented. Therefore, the reader is encouraged to stay abreast of new developments. Drug dosage and administration have been checked before publication, however, we recommend the reader always check product information for changes in dosage or administration before administering any drugs.

Skidmore-Roth Publishing, Inc.
400 Inverness Drive South, Suite 260
Englewood, Colorado 80112
(800) 825-3150
www.skidmore-roth.com

ISBN 1-56930-090-9

Acknowledgments

The Author would like to thank numerous individuals for their assistance in the development of this handbook. In their own way, their contribution helped to produce this book.

Rae Robertson and Lynne Kendall, Editors, Skidmore-Roth Publishing for their support and expertise, and for taking over this project after we had already started.

Kathleen Donley, RPh; Joe Snoke, RPh and pharmacy staff of Akron General Medical Center Department of Pharmacy for their assistance in creating the prescription medication section.

Chris Allen, RN, CDE of the Diabetic Center at Akron General Medical Center.

The Akron General Medical Center Paramedic Education staff of Denny Brawley, John Carney, Don Fobean, Les Gaiser and Mike Reed for "picking up the slack" while I worked on this book and their unknowing contributions while I watched them teach our students.

The Department of Emergency Medicine at Akron General Medical Center as well as all departments, including the physicians, nurses, and staff who help train and educate paramedics.

Carla Kachmar and the administration at Akron General Medical Center for their support and encouragement.

Chrissy Shepper for typing much of the manuscript and having to read my handwriting.

The men and women at Hudson Volunteer Emergency Medical Services for allowing me to work with them.

The reviewers, for their time and much needed input to the creation of this book, Dr. Thomas Elson for his expert knowledge of medicine, his time and energy into the review of this book, and his allowing me my own creative space.

And special recognition to Lory Shepper, administrative secretary for the Paramedic Education Program at Akron General Medical Center for her time, typing skills, unbelievable patience, computer wizardry, manuscript preparation (draft after draft), and her ability to keep everything else running smoothly in the paramedic program while this "project" moved forward to completion.

Consultants

Thomas J. Elson, M.D., F.A.C.E.P
Medical Director
A.G.M.C. Paramedic Education Program
Akron, Ohio

Reviewers

Jonathon D. Apfelbaum, M.D.
Emergency Physician
E.M.S. Fellow
Carolinas Medical Center
Charlotte, North Carolina

Annie Dorchak-Walters, E.M.T.-P
Former E.M.S. Educator
North Suburban Medical Center
Thornton, Colorado

Mary Ann Forrester, R.N., B.S.N., C.C.R.N, E.M.T.
Children's Hospital Medical Center of Akron
Akron, Ohio

James Holbrook, E.M.T.-P, M.A.
Program Director
Crafton Hills College
Yucaipa, California

Berni T. Martin, R.N., C.E.N., C.C.R.N.
Hudson, Ohio

Melissa B. Robinson, R.N., B.S.H., E.M.T.-P
Paramedic Coordinator
Brevard Community College
Coca, Florida

TABLE OF CONTENTS

Quick Reference Medication Dosages for Adults and Pediatrics

Adult Emergency Medication Dosages

MEDICATION	INDICATIONS, ROUTES and DOSAGES
Activated Charcoal (Instachar)	<u>Ingested poisons:</u> 50-100 grams mixed with a glass of water or juice to form a slurry. Do not mix with milk. Instruct the patient to drink the slurry.
Adenosine: (Adenocard)	<u>SVT:</u> 6 mg rapid IV push given over 1-2 seconds. May repeat within 2 minutes at 12 mg if not converted. May repeat the 12 mg dose one time.
Albuterol (Proventil)	<u>Asthma/respiratory distress:</u> 3 ml (2.5 mg) mixed in 2 ml NS by nebulization until medication is gone. May repeat up to 3 total doses.
Ammonia Inhalant	<u>Syncope:</u> 1 ampule placed 2 to 3 inches from nostrils
Amyl Nitrate (Vaporole) (In a Lilly cyanide kit)	<u>Cyanide poisoning:</u> 0.3 ml ampules inhaled by the patient and repeated until sodium nitrate IV is available
Aspirin (ASA)	<u>Cardiac chest pain:</u> 160 to 325 mg orally. Have the patient chew the tablets.
Atropine Sulfate	<u>Bradycardias</u> - IV: 0.5 mg initial dose, may repeat at 1.0 mg

MEDICATION	INDICATIONS, ROUTES and DOSAGES
	every 3-5 minutes up to a total of 2.5 mg or 0.03 mg/Kg
	Asystole or bradycardiac PEA - IV: 1 mg IV every 3-5 minutes up to 3 mg or 0.04 mg/Kg
	Endotracheal tube (ETT): 1-2 mg in 10 ml of NS.
	Organophosphate poisoning - IV: 2-10 mg repeated until the patient's respiratory status improves
Bretylium Tosylate (Bretylol)	Pulseless ventricular tachycardia or fibrillation: 5 mg/Kg IV repeated at 10 mg/Kg every 5 minutes up to 35 mg/Kg
	Ventricular tachycardia with a pulse: mix 5-10 mg/Kg in 50 ml NS and infuse over 10 minutes using a 10 gtt/ml IV administration set running at 50 gtt/min
	IV infusion for post conversion: 1-2 mg/min
	IV infusion mixture: 500 mg in 250 ml NS or 1 gram in 500 ml NS to equal a 2 mg/ml concentration

MEDICATION	INDICATIONS, ROUTES and DOSAGES
Calcium Chloride	Antidote for calcium channel blocker overdose, hypocalcemia/hyperkalemia: 2-4 mg/Kg of a 10% solution slow IV push. May be repeated at 10 minute intervals.
Dexamethasone (Decadron)	Allergic reactions, asthma: 0.1-0.25 mg/Kg IV slow push
50% Dextrose (D50)	Hypoglycemia: 50 ml of 50% Dextrose (25 Gm). May be repeated if there is no response or a minimal response is noted in marked hypoglycemia.
Diazepam (Valium)	Seizures: 2-10 mg IV until the seizure stops. Anxiety and sedation: 2-5 mg IV.
Diphenhydramine (Benadryl)	Anaphylaxis: 1 mg/Kg up to 25 mg IVP. 10–50 mg deep IM.
Dopamine (Dopastat, Intropin)	Hypotension: 2-20 mcg/Kg/min by IV infusion. (Dopaminergic: 1-2 mcg/kg/min; Beta: 2-10 mcg/Kg/min; Alpha: over 10 mcg/Kg/min) Generally, dopamine is started at 2-5

MEDICATION

INDICATIONS, ROUTES and DOSAGES

mcg/Kg/min (30 gtts/min) and titrated to a systolic blood pressure of 90 or 100 mmHg.

IV infusion mixture: 200 mg in 250 ml NS or 400 mg in 500 ml NS to equal a 800 mcg/ml concentration. Or, 400 mg in 250 ml NS to equal a 1600 mcg/ml concentration.

(See Adult Dopamine Infusion Chart, pg. 13)

Epinephrine 1:10,000
(Adrenalin)

Cardiac Arrest including Ventricular Fibrillation or Pulseless Ventricular Tachycardia, Asystole and PEA: 1.0 mg IV push repeated every 3-5 min.

Anaphylaxis refractory to SQ 1:1,000 epinephrine: 0.01 ml/kg (0.001 mg/kg) 1:10,000 IV slow push up to 5 ml (0.5 mg).

Epinephrine 1:1,000
(Adrenalin)

Anaphylaxis and asthma: (0.01 mg/Kg) usually 0.3-0.5 mg (0.3-0.5 ml) subcuta- neously

ETT: add 2.0 mg epinephrine in 8 ml normal saline

MEDICATION	INDICATIONS, ROUTES and DOSAGES
	<u>IV infusion:</u> 2 -10 mcg/min (start at 30 gtt/min and titrate to effect) by mixing 1 mg in 500 ml NS.
	<u>Repeat doses for cardiac arrest:</u> 0.1 mg/Kg IV or 5 mg IV
Flumazenil (Romazicon, Mazicon)	<u>Benzodiazepine overdoses:</u> 0.2 mg IV slow push over 30 seconds. If the desired changes are not achieved in 1-2 minutes, repeat at 0.3 mg IV over 30 seconds to a maximum dose of 3.0 mg.
Furosemide (Lasix)	<u>Pulmonary edema:</u> 1 mg/Kg slow IV push
Glucagon	<u>Hypoglycemia:</u> 1–2 mg deep IM, IV push.
Ipecac	<u>Emetic:</u> 30 ml (2 tablespoons) followed by several glasses of water.
Isoproterenol (Isuprel, Isopro)	<u>Refractory bradycardia, Torsades de Pointe:</u> 2-10 mcg/min IV infusion titrated to effect.
	<u>IV infusion mixture:</u> 1 mg in 500 ml NS to equal a 2 mcg/ml concentration

MEDICATION	INDICATIONS, ROUTES and DOSAGES
Lidocaine (Xylocaine)	<u>Pulseless VT or VF:</u> 1.5 mg/kg IV repeated every 3 to 5 minutes up to a total of 3 mg/Kg.
	<u>PVC's or VT with a pulse:</u> 1-1.5 mg/Kg IV repeated at 0.75 mg/Kg IV every 3 to 5 minutes up to a total of 3 mg/kg.
	<u>Maintenance infusion:</u> 2-4 mg/min. (Give half of this for patients with an acute MI, CHF, shock, age greater than 70, or those with hepatic dysfunction.)
	<u>ETT:</u> 2 times the IV dose
	<u>IV infusion mixture:</u> 1 gram in 250 ml NS or 2 grams in 500 ml NS to equal a 4 mg/ml concentration.
Magnesium Sulfate	<u>Eclampsia:</u> 2–4 grams diluted in 100 ml NS given IV slow push or by infusion
	<u>Torsades and refractory ventricular fibrillation and ventricular tachycardia:</u> 1-2 grams IV slow push.
Meperidine (Demerol)	<u>Pain relief:</u> 1 mg/kg IV titrated to effect.

MEDICATION	INDICATIONS, ROUTES and DOSAGES
Methylprednisolone (Solu-medrol)	<u>Anaphylatic shock, acute asthma:</u> 2 mg/Kg or 125 mg doses given IV. <u>Spinal cord injury:</u> 30 mg/Kg loading dose given IV.
Midazolam (Versed)	<u>Seizures, sedation prior to cardioversion:</u> 0.5 mg up to 5 mg slow IV or 5 mg deep IM titrated to effect. Consider lower doses for patients with respiratory diseases or those older than 60 years of age.
Morphine Sulfate (Duramorph)	<u>Pain relief, pulmonary edema:</u> 1-3 mg slow IV every 5-30 minutes titrated to effect. Use lower doses in the elderly.
Naloxone (Narcan)	<u>Narcotic overdoses:</u> 2.0 mg IV/IM/SC repeated every 2-3 minutes as necessary up to a total of 10 mg. <u>ETT:</u> 4 mg added to NS for a total volume of 10 ml in a syringe
Nitroglycerin	<u>Cardiac chest pain:</u> Tablets: 0.3 mg (1/200 gr) or 0.4 mg (1/150 gr) sublingual every 5

MEDICATION	INDICATIONS, ROUTES and DOSAGES

minutes up to three tablets or complete relief.

<u>Spray:</u> 1 sublingual spray every 5 minutes up to 3 sprays or complete relief.

<u>IV Infusion:</u> 5-10 mcg/min (3-6 gtts/min using a 60 gtt/ml IV administration set) slowly titrating to pain relief or until hypotension ensues.

<u>IV infusion mixture:</u> 5 ml (25 mg) in 250 ml NS to equal a 100 mcg/ml concentration.

(See Adult Nitroglycerin Infusion Chart, pg. 15.)

Nitrous Oxide
(Nitronox)

<u>Pain relief:</u> Self administration by mask. Once patient has had enough and the pain is relieved, the patient will drop the mask and begin to breathe room air.

Oxytocin
(Pitocin)

<u>Postpartum bleeding:</u> IV infusion of 10 units in 500 ml NS starting at 20-40 milliunits per minute titrated to effect.

Procainamide
(Pronestyl, Procan)

<u>Ventricular and supraventricular tachycardias:</u> IV loading infusion: 20 mg/min by

MEDICATION	INDICATIONS, ROUTES and DOSAGES
	adding 1 gram (1 g/10 ml) to 40 ml NS to equal 20 mg/ml. Infuse using a 60 gtt/ml IV administration set at 60 gtts/min. Infuse the procainamide until either the arrhythmia is suppressed, hypotension develops, the QRS complex widens by 50%, or a total of 17 mg/Kg has been given.
	Maintenance infusion: 1-4 mg/min.
	IV infusion mixture: 1 gram in 250 ml NS or 2 grams in 500 ml NS to equal a 4 mg/ml concentration.
Prochlorperazine (Compazine)	Nausea and vomiting: 5-10 mg IV/IM watching for hypotension. In older patients consider half doses.
Proparacaine (Alcaine, Ophthaine)	Topical eye anesthetic: 1-2 drops in the affected eye.
Sodium Bicarbonate	Acidosis, TCA overdoses: 1 mEq/Kg IV repeating half (1/2) the initial dose every 10 minutes.

MEDICATION	INDICATIONS, ROUTES and DOSAGES
	Crush injuries: add 50 ml (50 mEq) in 1000 ml NS or 0.45% NS and infuse.
Sodium Nitrate (In a Lilly cyanide kit)	Cyanide poisoning: 10 ml (300 mg) IV over 20 minutes watching for hypotension.
Sodium Thiosulfate (In a Lilly cyanide kit)	Cyanide poisoning: 50 ml (12.5 grams) IV over 20 minutes.
Tetracaine (Pontocaine)	Topical eye anesthetic: 1-2 drops in the affected eye.
Thiamine (Betalin)	Thiamine replacement: 100 mg IV slow push.
Verapamil (Calan, Isoptin)	Atrial fibrillation/flutter: 2.5 to 5 mg initial dose slow IV over 1-3 minutes. May repeat at 5-10 mg every 15-30 minutes. Patients over 70 years of age should receive smaller doses (2-4 mg) over a longer period of time (3-4 minutes).

More information about each drug can be found in Section 13 under Emergency Medication Information.

Adult Dopamine Infusion Chart

Locate the weight across the top of the chart and the mcg/kg/min rate on the left.

Where the weight column and the mcg/kg/min row intersect is the ml/hour rate when using an infusion pump, or the gtts/min rate using a 60 gtt/ml IV administration set.

Round ml/hour, gtts/min rate to the nearest even number.

Rate table for solution of dopamine mixed 400 mg in 500 ml or 200 mg in 250 ml normal saline. Concentration = 800 mcg/ml

800 mcg/ml

Patient Weight (kg)

Rate in mcg/kg/min	50	55	60	65	70	75	80	85	90	95	100
1	3.8	4.1	4.5	4.9	5.3	5.6	6.0	6.4	6.8	7.1	7.5
2	7.5	8.3	9.0	9.8	10.5	11.3	12.0	12.8	13.5	14.3	15.0
2.5	9.4	10.3	11.3	12.2	13.1	14.1	15.0	15.9	16.9	17.8	18.8
3	11.3	12.4	13.5	14.6	15.8	16.9	18.0	19.1	20.3	21.4	22.5
4	15.0	16.5	18.0	19.5	21.0	22.5	24.0	25.5	27.0	28.5	30.0
5	18.8	20.6	22.5	24.4	26.3	28.1	30.0	31.9	33.8	35.6	37.5
6	22.5	24.8	27.0	29.3	31.5	33.8	36.0	38.3	40.5	42.8	45.0
7	26.3	28.9	31.5	34.1	36.8	39.4	42.0	44.6	47.3	49.9	52.5
7.5	28.1	30.9	33.8	36.6	39.4	42.2	45.0	47.8	50.6	53.4	56.3
8	30.0	33.0	36.0	39.0	42.0	45.0	48.0	51.0	54.0	57.0	60.0
10	37.5	41.3	45.0	48.8	52.5	56.3	60.0	63.8	67.5	71.3	75.0
12	45.0	49.5	54.0	58.5	63.0	67.5	72.0	76.5	81.0	85.5	90.0

Rate table for solution of dopamine mixed 400 mg in 250 ml normal saline. Concentration = 1600 mcg/ml

1600 mcg/ml

Patient Weight (kg)

Rate in mcg/kg/min	50	55	60	65	70	75	80	85	90	95	100
1	1.9	2.1	2.3	2.4	2.6	2.8	3.0	3.2	3.4	3.6	3.8
2	3.8	4.1	4.5	4.9	5.3	5.6	6.0	6.4	6.8	7.1	7.5
2.5	4.7	5.2	5.6	6.1	6.6	7.0	7.5	8.0	8.4	8.9	9.4
3	5.6	6.2	6.8	7.3	7.9	8.4	9.0	9.6	10.1	10.7	11.3
4	7.5	8.3	9.0	9.8	10.5	11.3	12.0	12.8	13.5	14.3	15.0
5	9.4	10.3	11.3	12.2	13.1	14.1	15.0	15.9	16.9	17.8	18.8
6	11.3	12.4	13.5	14.6	15.8	16.9	18.0	19.1	20.3	21.4	22.5
7	13.1	14.4	15.8	17.1	18.4	19.7	21.0	22.3	23.6	24.9	26.3
7.5	14.1	15.5	16.9	18.3	19.7	21.1	22.5	23.9	25.3	26.7	28.1
8	15.0	16.5	18.0	19.5	21.0	22.5	24.0	25.5	27.0	28.5	30.0
10	18.8	20.6	22.5	24.4	26.3	28.1	30.0	31.9	33.8	35.6	37.5
12	22.5	24.8	27.0	29.3	31.5	33.8	36.0	38.3	40.5	42.8	45.0

Adult Nitroglycerin Infusion Chart

25 mg in 250 ml or 50 mg in 500 ml normal saline to equal 100 mcg/ml			50 mg in 250 ml or 100 mg in 500 ml nomal saline to equal 200 mcg/ml		
To Deliver:	Infusion Pump	60 gtt/ml IV Admin. Set	To Deliver:	Infusion Pump	60 gtt/ml IV Admin. Set
5 mcg/min =	3 cc/hr	3 gtts/min	10 mcg/min =	3 cc/hr	3 gtts/min
10 mcg/min=	6 cc/hr	6 gtts/min	20 mcg/min=	6 cc/hr	6 gtts/min
20 mcg/min=	12 cc/hr	12 gtts/min	30 mcg/min=	9 cc/hr	9 gtts/min
30 mcg/min=	18 cc/hr	18 gtts/min	40 mcg/min=	12 cc/hr	12 gtts/min
40 mcg/min=	24 cc/hr	24 gtts/min	50 mcg/min=	15 cc/hr	15 gtts/min
50 mcg/min=	30 cc/hr	30 gtts/min	60 mcg/min=	18 cc/hr	18 gtts/min
60 mcg/min=	36 cc/hr	36 gtts/min	70 mcg/min=	21 cc/hr	21 gtts/min
70 mcg/min=	42 cc/hr	42 gtts/min	80 mcg/min=	24 cc/hr	24 gtts/min
80 mcg/min=	48 cc/hr	48 gtts/min	90 mcg/min=	27 cc/hr	27 gtts/min
90 mcg/min=	54 cc/hr	54 gtts/min	100 mcg/min=	30 cc/hr	30 gtts/min
100 mcg/min=	60 cc/hr	60 gtts/min	110 mcg/min=	33 cc/hr	33 gtts/min
110 mcg/min=	66 cc/hr	66 gtts/min	120 mcg/min=	36 cc/hr	36 gtts/min
120 mcg/min=	72 cc/hr	72 gtts/min	130 mcg/min=	39 cc/hr	39 gtts/min
130 mcg/min=	78 cc/hr	78 gtts/min	140 mcg/min=	42 cc/hr	42 gtts/min
140 mcg/min=	84 cc/hr	84 gtts/min	150 mcg/min=	45 cc/hr	45 gtts/min
150 mcg/min=	90 cc/hr	90 gtts/min	160 mcg/min=	48 cc/hr	48 gtts/min
160 mcg/min=	96 cc/hr	96 gtts/min	170 mcg/min=	51 cc/hr	51 gtts/min
170 mcg/min=	102 cc/hr	102 gtts/min	180 mcg/min=	54 cc/hr	54 gtts/min
180 mcg/min=	108 cc/hr	108 gtts/min	190 mcg/min=	57 cc/hr	57 gtts/min
190 mcg/min=	114 cc/hr	114 gtts/min	200 mcg/min=	60 cc/hr	60 gtts/min
200 mcg/min=	120 cc/hr	120 gtts/min			

Pediatric Emergency Medication Dosages

MEDICATION	INDICATIONS, ROUTES and DOSAGES
Activated Charcoal (Instachar)	Ingested poisons: 1 gram/Kg mixed with a glass of water to form a slurry. Do not mix with milk. Have the patient drink the slurry.
Adenosine (Adenocard)	SVT: 0.1 mg/Kg (max 6 mg) rapid IV and IO. May repeat within 2 minutes at 0.2 mg/Kg (max 12 mg).
Albuterol (Proventil)	Asthma, respiratory distress: 2 years of age and older: 3 ml (2.5 mg) in 2 ml NS by nebulization until medication is gone. May need to repeat up to 3 total doses. Less than 2 years of age: 1.5 ml (1.25 mg) in 2 ml NS by nebulization until medication is gone. May need to repeat up to 3 total doses.

MEDICATION	INDICATIONS, ROUTES and DOSAGES

Amyl Nitrate
(Vaporole)
(In Lilly cyanide kit)

Cyanide poisoning: 0.3 ml ampules inhaled by the patient and repeated until sodium nitrate IV is available.

Atropine Sulfate

Bradycardia (after no response to 2-3 rounds of epinephrine): 0.02 mg/Kg IV, IO (minimum IV, IO dose 0.1 mg).
Children less than 5 years old: maximum single dose 0.5 mg, maximum total dose 1.0 mg.
Children over 5 years old: maximum single dose 1.0 mg, maximum total dose 2.0 mg.
ETT: 0.04 to 0.06 mg/Kg (minimum ETT dose 0.15 mg).

Bretylium Tosylate
(Bretylol)

Pulseless ventricular tachycardia or ventricular fibrillation: 5 mg/Kg IV repeated at 10 mg/Kg every 5 minutes up to 35 mg/Kg total dose.
Ventricular tachycardia with a pulse: mix 5-10 mg/Kg in 50 ml NS and infuse over 10 minutes using a 10 gtt/ml IV administration set infusing at 50 gtt/min.

MEDICATION	INDICATIONS, ROUTES and DOSAGES

<u>IV maintenance infusion for post conversion:</u> 1-2 mg/min.
<u>IV infusion mixture:</u> 500 mg in 250 ml NS or 1 gram in 500 ml NS to equal a 2 mg/ml concentration.

Calcium Chloride

<u>Antidote for calcium channel blocker overdose:</u> 5-7 mg/Kg of a 10% solution slow IV push, IO. May be repeated at 10 minute intervals.

Dexamethasone
(Decadron)

<u>Allergic reactions, asthma:</u> 0.1-0.25 mg/Kg IV slow push.

50% Dextrose
(D50)

<u>Hypoglycemia:</u>
<u>Neonate to 1 year:</u> 2-4 ml/Kg of a 10% dextrose solution. To make a 10% dextrose solution, squirt out 40 ml of D50 and replace it with 40 ml of normal saline or sterile water.
<u>1 year to 10 years:</u> 2-4 ml/Kg of a 25% dextrose solution. To make a 25% dextrose solution, squirt out 25 ml of D50 and replace it with 25 ml of normal saline or sterile water.

MEDICATION	INDICATIONS, ROUTES and DOSAGES
Diazepam (Valium)	Seizures: IV: 0.2-0.3 mg/Kg up to 5 mg slow IV push. Rectal: 0.5 mg/Kg up to 10 mg.
Diphenhydramine (Benadryl)	Anaphylaxis: 0.5 mg to 1 mg/Kg up to 25 mg slow IV or IM.
Dopamine (Dopastat, Intropin)	Hypotension: IV infusion: 2-20 mcg/Kg/min. Starting dose: 5-10 mcg/Kg/min. IV infusion mixture: add 100 mg (2.5 ml of a 40 mg/ml solution) dopamine into 250 ml NS or 200 mg (5 ml of a 40 mg/ml solution) into 500 ml NS (400 mcg/ml concentration). Using a 60 gtt/ml IV administration set, start the drip rate off at the patient's weight in Kg which will start the infusion at 6.7 mcg/Kg/min. **(See Pediatric Dopamine Infusion Chart, pg. 24.)**
Epinephrine 1:10,000 (Adrenalin)	Pulseless arrest: epinephrine 1:10,000 is given as the first dose, using 0.1 ml/Kg (0.01 mg/Kg) IV or IO.

| MEDICATION | INDICATIONS, ROUTES and DOSAGES |

(1:1,000 epinephrine is used in subsequent doses.) <u>Brady cardia</u>, 1:10,000 is given 0.1 mL/Kg (0.01 mg/Kg) every 3-5 minutes.

Epinephrine 1:1,000
(Adrenalin)

<u>Anaphylaxis and asthma:</u> 0.01 ml/Kg (0.01 mg/Kg) up to 0.3 ml total dose. <u>Repeat dosages in cardiac arrest:</u> 0.1 ml/Kg (0.1 mg/Kg) IVP, IO, ETT every 3 to 5 minutes. <u>IV infusion:</u> 0.05-2 mcg/Kg/min (start at 0.1-0.3 mcg/Kg/min and titrate to effect). IV infusion mixtures: <u>Children 2-20 Kg:</u> Add 3 mg (3 ml) into 250 ml NS (12 mcg/ml concentration). Using a 60 gtt/ml IV administration set starting the drip rate off at the patient's weight in Kg to administer the infusion at 0.2 mcg/kg/min and titrate to effect. <u>Children 21-40 Kg:</u> Add 6 mg (6 ml) into 250 ml NS (24 mcg/ml concentration). Using a 60 gtt/ml IV administration set starting the drip rate off at half (1/2) the patent's weight in Kg to

MEDICATION	INDICATIONS, ROUTES and DOSAGES
	administer the infusion at 0.2 mcg/kg/min and titrate to effect.

(See Pediatric Epinephrine Infusion Chart, pg. 25.)

Furosemide
(Lasix)

Pulmonary edema: 1 mg/Kg slow IVP (maximum dose = 20 mg).

Glucagon

Hypoglycemia: 0.03 mg/Kg up to 1 mg deep IM.

Ipecac

Emetic: Children less than 1 year of age: 5-10 ml (1-2 tea spoons) follow by as much water as possible. Children 1-15 years of age: 15 ml (one tablespoon) followed by several glasses of water (do not use milk or carbonated beverages).

Lidocaine
(Xylocaine)

Ventricular arrhythmias: 1 mg/Kg IV/IO q 10-15 minutes IV infusion dosage range: 20-50 mcg/Kg/min.
IV infusion mixture: add 300 mg into 250 ml normal saline to equal a 1200 mcg/ml concentration. Using a 60 gtt/ml IV administration set,

MEDICATION	INDICATIONS, ROUTES and DOSAGES
	start the infusion off at the patient's weight in Kg to administer the infusion at 20 mcg/Kg/min and titrate to effect. **(See Pediatric Lidocaine Infusion Chart, pg. 27.)**
Meperidine (Demerol)	<u>Pain relief:</u> IV, IO: 1 mg/Kg up to 50 mg slow IV/IO.
Methylprednisolone (Solu-medrol)	<u>Anaphylactic shock, acute asthma:</u> 1-2 mg/Kg doses given IV. <u>Spinal cord injury:</u> 30 mg/Kg loading dose given IV.
Midazolam (Versed)	<u>Seizures:</u> 0.1-0.3 mg/Kg slow IV/IO, deep IM up to 5 mg
Morphine Sulfate (Duramorph)	<u>Pain relief:</u> 0.05-0.1 mg/Kg slow IV/IO.
Naloxone (Narcan)	<u>Narcotic overdoses:</u> 0.1 mg/Kg up to 2 mg IV/IO/IM/SC. May repeat in 5 minutes. <u>ETT:</u> 2-3 times the IV dose.

MEDICATION	INDICATIONS, ROUTES and DOSAGES
Nitrous Oxide (Nitronox)	Self-administration by mask. Once patient has had enough and the pain is relieved, the patient will drop the mask and begin to breathe room air.
Proparacaine (Alcaine, Ophthaine)	Topical eye anesthetic: 1-2 drops in the affected eye.
Sodium Bicarbonate	Acidosis, TCP overdoses: 1 year and older: 1 mEq/Kg IV (can repeat every 10 minutes) using a 8.4% solution. Newborn to 1 year old: 1-2 mEq/Kg IV (can repeat every 10 minutes using a 4.2% solution). To make a 4.2% solution, squirt out 25 ml from an 8.4% solution and replace it with 25 ml sterile water.
Tetracaine (Protocaine)	Topical eye anesthetic: 1-2 drops in the affected eye.

More information about each drug can be found in Section 13 under Emergency Medication Information.

Pediatric Dopamine Infusion Chart

Dosage range for a dopamine infusion 5-20 mcg/Kg/minute. Starting dosage range is 5-10 mcg/Kg/minute. Mix 100 mg (2.5 ml of 40 mg/ml) in 250 ml normal saline to give a 400 mcg/ml concentration. Using a 60 gtt/ml IV administration set, the starting drip rate will be the same as the patient's weight in kilograms to administer an initial dose of 6.7 mcg/Kg/minute and titrate to effect. Round the drip rates up to whole numbers.

Starting Drip Rate **100 mg/250 ml = 400 mcg/ml**
To Give

DRIP RATE

Pt Wt in Kg	Starting Drip Rate	6.7 mcg/Kg/minute	8.3	10	11.7	13.3	15	16.7	18.3	20
2	2	2	-	3	-	4	-	5	-	6
4	4	4	5	6	7	8	9	10	11	12
6	6	6	7.5	9	10.5	12	13.5	15	16.5	18
8	8	8	10	12	14	16	18	20	22	24
10	10	10	12.5	15	17.5	20	22.5	25	27.5	30
12	12	12	15	18	21	24	27	30	33	36
14	14	14	17.5	21	24.5	28	31.5	35	38.5	42
16	16	16	20	24	28	32	36	40	44	48
18	18	18	22.5	27	31.5	36	40.5	45	51.5	54
20	20	20	25	30	35	40	45	50	55	60
22	22	22	27.5	33	38.5	44	49.5	55	60.5	66
24	24	24	30	36	42	48	54	60	66	72
26	26	26	32.5	39	45.5	52	58.5	65	71.5	78
28	28	28	35	42	49	56	63	70	77	84
30	30	30	37.5	45	52.5	60	67.5	75	82.5	90
32	32	32	40	48	56	64	72	80	88	96
34	34	34	42.5	51	59.5	68	76.5	85	93.5	102
36	36	36	45	54	63	72	81	90	99	108
38	38	38	47.5	57	66.5	76	85.5	95	104.5	114
40	40	40	50	60	70	80	90	100	110	120

Pediatric Epinephrine Infusion Chart

Epinephrine dosage range 0.05-2.0 mcg/Kg/minute
Starting dosage range 0.1-0.3 mcg/Kg/minute

1. Determine the child's weight in kilograms.
2. Mix epinephrine according to chart below.

Pt. Wt. in Kg	Mixture	Starting drip rate using 60 gtt/ml IV set up
2-20 Kg (4.4-44 lbs)	3 mg in 250 ml NS	Pt. wt. in Kg to start at 0.2 mcg/Kg/min
22-40 Kg (48-88 lbs)	6 mg in 250 ml NS	1/2 Pt. wt. in Kg to start at 0.2 mcg/Kg/min

Starting Drip Rate　　　　**3 mg/250 ml = 12 mcg/ml**

To give for a 2-20 Kg child

Pt Wt in Kg	DRIP RATE	mcg/kg/min									
		0.2	0.4	0.6	0.8	1.0	1.2	1.4	1.6	1.8	2.0
2	2	2	4	6	8	10	12	14	16	18	20
4	4	4	8	12	16	20	24	28	32	36	40
6	6	6	12	18	24	30	36	42	18	54	60
8	8	8	16	24	32	40	48	56	64	72	80
10	10	10	20	30	40	50	60	70	80	90	100
12	12	12	24	36	48	60	72	84	96	108	120
14	14	14	28	42	56	70	84	98	112	126	140
16	16	16	32	48	64	80	96	112	128	144	160
18	18	18	36	54	72	90	108	126	144	162	180
20	20	20	40	60	80	100	120	140	160	180	200

Starting Drip Rate		6 mg/250 ml = 24 mcg/ml									
		To give for a 22-40 Kg child									
Pt Wt in Kg		mcg/kg/min									
		0.2	0.4	0.6	0.8	1.0	1.2	1.4	1.6	1.8	2.0
22	11	11	22	33	44	55	66	77	88	99	110
24	12	12	24	36	48	60	72	84	96	108	120
26	13	13	26	39	52	65	78	91	104	117	130
28	14	14	28	41	56	70	84	98	112	126	140
30	15	15	30	45	60	75	90	105	120	135	150
32	16	16	32	48	64	80	96	112	128	144	160
34	17	17	34	51	68	85	102	119	136	153	170
36	18	18	36	54	72	90	108	126	144	162	180
38	19	19	38	57	76	95	114	133	152	171	190
40	20	20	40	60	80	100	120	140	160	180	200

DRIP RATE

Pediatric Lidocaine Infusion Chart

The dosage range for a lidocaine infusion is 20-50 mcg/Kg/minute. The starting dose is 20 mcg/Kg/minute. Mix 300 mg (30 ml of 10 mg/ml) in 250 ml normal saline to give a 1200 mcg/ml concentration. Using a 60 gtt/ml IV administration set, the starting drip rate will be the same as the patient's weight in kilograms to administer an initial dose of 20 mcg/Kg/minute and titrate to effect. Round any drip rates up to a whole number.

300 mg/250 ml = 1200 mcg/ml

Pt Wt in Kg	Starting Drip Rate	To Give mcg/Kg/minute						
		20	25	30	35	40	45	50
2	2	2	-	3	-	4	-	5
4	4	4	5	6	7	8	9	10
6	6	6	7.5	9	10.5	12	13.5	15
8	8	8	10	12	14	16	18	20
10	10	10	12.5	15	17.5	20	22.5	25
12	12	12	15	18	21	24	27	30
14	14	14	17.5	21	24.5	28	31.5	35
16	16	16	20	24	28	32	36	40
18	18	18	22.5	27	31.5	36	40.5	45
20	20	20	25	30	35	40	45	50
22	22	22	27.5	33	38.5	44	49.5	55
24	24	24	30	36	42	48	54	60
26	26	26	32.5	39	45.5	52	58.5	65
28	28	28	35	42	49	56	63	70
30	30	30	37.5	45	52.5	60	67.5	75
32	32	32	40	48	56	64	72	80
34	34	34	42.5	51	59.5	68	76.5	85
36	36	36	45	54	63	72	81	90
38	38	38	47.5	57	66.5	76	85.5	95
40	40	40	50	60	70	80	90	100

(DRIP RATE)

EKG's and Cardiology

Limb Lead Placement

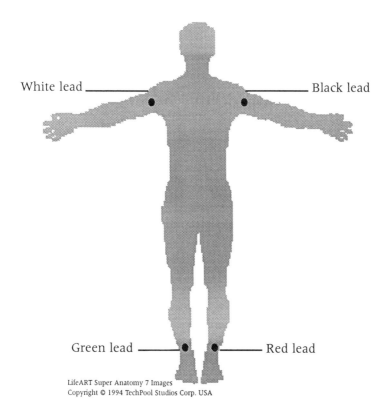

White lead —————————— Black lead

Green lead —————— Red lead

LifeART Super Anatomy 7 Images
Copyright © 1994 TechPool Studios Corp. USA

Lead	Limb
White	Right shoulder/arm
Black	Left shoulder/arm
Red	Left leg
Green (ground)	Right leg

Limb Lead Views

	Bipolar Limb Lead		Unipolar (Augmented Voltage) Limb Leads		
Lead	Positive	Negative	Lead	Positive	"Negative" is in between
I	Black	White	AVF	Red	White and Black
II	Red	White	AVL	Black	White and Red
III	Red	Black	AVR	White	Black and Red
	Ground is always green			Ground is always green	

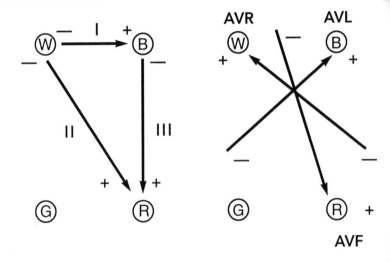

Bipolar leads use a "true" negative lead.

Unipolar leads "assume" a negative lead opposite the positive lead.

Precordial Chest Leads

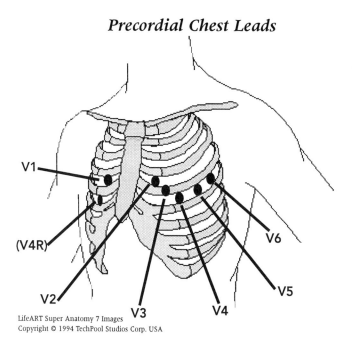

LifeART Super Anatomy 7 Images
Copyright © 1994 TechPool Studios Corp. USA

Precordial (unipolar) Chest Lead Placement

Lead	Positive Lead	"Negative Lead"
V1	Right sternal border, 4th intercostal space	
V2	Left sternal border, 4th intercostal space	Assumed to be on the opposite side of the thorax that the positive lead is looking toward.
V3	Forming a straight line between V2 and V4	
V4	Left mid clavicular line, 5th intercostal space	
V5	Left anterior axillary line, 5th intercostal space	
V6	Left mid axillary line, 5th intercostal space	
(V4R)	Right mid clavicular line, 5th intercostal space (used when looking at the right ventrical)	

Parameters for Interpretation of Cardiac Rhythms

Are there P waves for every QRS wave?

Are there QRS waves for every P wave?

Is the rhythm regular?

If irregular, is it regularly irregular or irregularly irregular?

What is the rate?

What is the PR interval? (normal - 0.12 to 0.20 seconds)

Is the PR interval constant or does it vary?

What is the length of the QRS complex? (normal - 0.04 to 0.12 seconds)

Determining Various Supraventricular Rhythms
having a narrow QRS (0.12 or less)

Heart Rate	Positive P Wave in Lead II	Negative P Wave in Lead II	P Wave Unknown in Lead II
<40	SB	JB	JB
40-60	SB	JR	JR
60-100	SR	JR	AJR
100-160	ST	JT	JT
160-220	AT	JT	SVT

SB	=	Sinus Bradycardia
JB	=	Junctional Bradycardia
SR	=	Sinus Rhythm
ST	=	Sinus Tachycardia
AT	=	Atrial Tachycardia
JT	=	Junctional Tachycardia
AJR	=	Accelerated Junctional Rhythm

Interpretation of Heart Blocks

<u>AV Nodal Blocks</u>

Ask the following questions:

Does the PR interval vary?

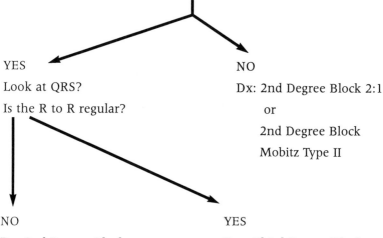

YES

Look at QRS?

Is the R to R regular?

NO

Dx: 2nd Degree Block 2:1

      or

    2nd Degree Block

    Mobitz Type II

NO

Dx: 2nd Degree Block

    Mobitz Type I

YES

Dx: Third Degree Block

    (The P to P will also

    be regular with no

    relationship to the QRS)

EKG Terminology and Definitions

Term	Definition
Ischemia	A decrease in blood flow and oxygen to a portion of the cardiac muscle causing cellular hypoxia. Onset of ischemia occurs seconds after diminished blood flow begins.
Injury	Ischemic myocardial muscle begins to die within minutes of diminished blood flow. Injury occurs between 20 and 40 minutes after the initial ischemic event. If blood flow can be restored, the myocardial muscle may be salvaged.
Infarction	Death of the myocardial muscle after prolonged ischemia. Occurs within minutes to hours after the initial decrease of blood flow and oxygen to the myocardial tissue.
Anatomically Contiguous Leads	Two or more different leads that look at the same area of the heart. Leads II, III and AVF all look at the inferior portion of the heart. EKG changes seen in these three leads support one another in that they are all seeing the same thing.

Reciprocal Changes

EKG changes that reflect what is occurring on the opposite side of the heart. As an example, the inferior leads (II, III, and AVF) will show reciprocal changes of a lateral wall ischemic event. If the lateral leads are showing ST segment depression (ischemia), it would be expected to see some ST segment elevation (reciprocal) in the inferior leads (because they are looking at the lateral wall from the opposite side). More than likely, there will be some reciprocal changes in the other leads as well since all leads are looking at the heart simultaneously.

Significant EKG Changes

EKG changes that strongly support the probability of myocardial muscle damage when looking at multiple contiguous leads.

Multiple Lead Changes

Corresponding contiguous leads which are all showing EKG changes in their respective areas of the heart. These changes indicate that both areas may be affected by loss of blood flow. Changes seen in V1 and V2 (septal), as well as in V3 and V4 (anterior) may be termed anteroseptal changes.

J Point Measurement

The point at which the wave form changes direction at the end of the QRS and the beginning of the ST segment. The J point is used as the reference point for ST segment changes.

EKG Changes Seen in Ischemia, Injury, and Infarction

EKG changes that are seen in two or more contiguous leads (excluding paced rhythms, left ventricular hypertrophy, and bundle branch blocks) indicate the following:

Ischemia

ST segment **DEPRESSION** of 1 mm (one small box) or greater below the base line measured from the baseline to the J point. Horizontal or downward sloping ST segments from the start of J point are significant. T wave inversion or tall peaked T waves may also be present.

Injury

ST segment **ELEVATION** of 1 mm (one small box) or greater above the base line measured 0.04 seconds (one small box) past the J point is significant.

Infarction

Q WAVES that are 1 mm (0.04 seconds) in width or greater and have a height (depth) that is 25% the height of the R wave or greater, are considered significant (abnormal). Significant Q waves in the presence of ST segment and/or T wave changes as described above indicate an acute myocardial infarction (AMI).

What to Look for

Area of the Left Ventricle	Presence of ST Changes or Q Waves in Leads	Reciprocal Changes	Coronary Artery Most Likely Involved
Septal	V1 & V2	V5, V6	LAD
Anterior	V3 & V4	II, III, and AVF	LAD
Lateral	I, AVL, V5, V6	V1, V2 or II, III, and AVF	LAD, circumflex
Inferior	II, III, AVF	V2, V3	RCA
Posterior	Posterior leads V7, V8, V9 (not commonly used)	ST depression with large R waves in V1, V2, and possible V3, V4 (look for these changes)	Circumflex
Right Ventricle	Consider with Inferior lead changes. Look at lead V4R.		RCA

What Each Lead Views of the Left Ventricle

Lead	View	Reason
I, AVL, V5, V6	Left <u>lateral</u> wall	The positive electrode of each lead is on the left side of the chest wall and looks at the lateral wall of the left ventricle.
II, III, AVF	<u>Inferior</u> wall (Apex)	The positive electrode of each lead is at the bottom of the left ventricle and looks at the inferior wall of the left ventricle.
V1, V2	<u>Septal</u> or right wall of left ventricle and posterior wall (reciprocal)	The positive electrode of each lead is on the right side of the left ventricle looking at the interventricular septum which separates the right and left ventricle.
V3, V4	<u>Anterior</u> wall and possibly the posterior wall (reciprocal)	The positive electrode of each lead looks at the anterior wall of the left ventricle.

12 lead EKG paper prints the view of each lead in this format.

I	AVR	V1	V4
II	AVL	V2	V5
III	AVF	V3	V6

By looking for EKG changes that are consistent in these leads relative to these locations, ischemia, injury, or infarct patterns may be easily seen.

I Lateral	AVR (AVR is not viewed)	V1 Septal (Posterior Recip.)	V4 Anterior (Posterior Recip.)
II Inferior	AVL Lateral	V2 Septal (Posterior Recip.)	V5 Lateral
III Inferior	AVF Inferior	V3 Anterior (Posterior Recip.)	V6 Lateral

Zones of Myocardial Infarction

The diagrams below represent the heart.

The following leads usually represent the zones of myocardial muscle that are either ischemic, injured, or infarcted.

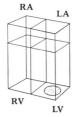

Inferior wall MI
Leads II, III, and
AVF

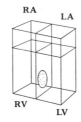

Septal wall MI
Leads V1 and V2

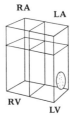

Lateral wall MI
Leads V5, V6, I,
and AVL

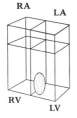

Anterior wall MI
Leads V3 and V4

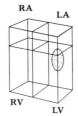

Posterior wall MI
Reciprocal changes
in leads V1, V2, V3,
and V4

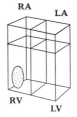

Right ventricular MI
If significant changes
are seen in inferior
leads II, III, and AVF,
look at lead V4R

Cardiac Pacemakers and Automatic Internal Cardioverter-Defibrillators (AICD's)

Cardiac Pacemakers

Cardiac pacemakers can either be permanent (implanted) or temporary. Permanent pacemakers have a generator and a battery pack which are most often implanted in the left chest wall below the clavicle. On occasion, the battery pack is implanted in the abdominal cavity. The pacemaker electrodes are fed into either the right atrium, right ventricle, or into both chambers (AV sequential), depending upon the patient's cardiac electrical conduction problems. Most of these pacemakers are "demand" pacers, which fire when the patient's own intrinsic heart rate drops below a set rate, usually around 72 beats per minute.

Problems Encountered with Pacemakers

1. Problems that occur with pacemakers are generally limited to the electrodes when they become dislodged.

2. Most batteries used in pacemakers are good for 10-14 years and the patient is usually well aware of the expiration date.

3. Newer pacers can be controlled or changed using a magnet waved over the pulse generator. Use of the magnet is not a prehospital procedure.

4. A pacemaker patient in cardiac arrest is treated like any other patient. If possible, avoid defibrillating through the pulse generator or battery pack to avoid damaging the devices. Due to their location in the chest or abdomen, this should not be a major concern.

5. When assessing a patient with a pacemaker, keep in mind that the pacemaker is only there to ensure an effective heart rate. These patients can still have acute myocardial infarction and more likely than not, the patient may have a history of past MI.

Automatic Implantable Cardioverter Defibrillators (AICD's)

AICD's are small implanted defibrillators used for high risk patients prone to ventricular tachycardia and/or ventricular fibrillation. The pulse generator is usually located in the abdominal cavity with wires running up to the sensor/electrode patches which are sutured around the ventricles of the heart. The sensors/electrodes monitor the patient's intrinsic heart rate and other parameters and in the presence of ventricular tachycardia or fibrillation, will cause the generator to charge and fire. Depending upon the type of AICD, the generator will defibrillate the heart 5 to 10 times over a 2 to 3 minute period looking for a sinus rhythm. If after the preset number of shocks have been reached with no change in the ventricular rhythm, the AICD will stop firing. The energy level during defibrillation is minimal (30 to 40 joules) and less than 2 joules reach the skin surface. With latex gloves on, prehospital personnel should not feel the electrical energy.

Interacting with Patients with AICD's

1. When encountering a patient with an AICD which is discharging, quickly attach your monitor/EKG electrodes to determine if the ventricular rhythm has converted.

2. Allow the AICD to complete its cycle before using the defibrillator paddles.

3. If the AICD stops firing after waiting thirty seconds, and the patient is still in ventricular tachycardia or fibrillation without a pulse, immediately defibrillate with the paddles and then follow standard ventricular treatment protocols.

4. Because of the insulated sensor/electrodes surrounding the heart, standard anterior-anterior paddle placement may not be effective. If this paddle placement is not working, switch to an anterior-posterior paddle placement.

Suggested Prehospital Cardiac Treatments (Adult)

Suggested Prehospital Treatment for Chest Pain and Possible Acute Myocardial Infarction (AMI)

Assess the patient

Establish an airway

Administer oxygen, 4 L/min via nasal cannula

Obtain a set of vital signs, pulse oximetry

Obtain a history from the patient

|

Apply the limb leads and determine the underlying rhythm

|

Establish an IV

|

If necessary, treat any arrhythmias appropriately

|

Consider giving aspirin, 160 to 325 mg PO

|

If the pain is not relieved by the oxygen
and patient is not hypotensive

|

Give nitroglycerin 0.3-0.4 mg sublingual every
5 minutes up to 3 tablets or sprays *

|

Consider morphine 1-3 mg IV slow push
for additional pain relief

|

Obtain a 12 lead EKG

|

Consult with the emergency department physician
on the EKG interpretation or transmit the EKG to the ED

|

Obtain history from the patient to consider
eligibility for thrombolytic therapy **

|

Continually reassure the patient

* If a right ventricular wall MI is possible, use nitroglycerin with caution. If the patient is hypotensive with a suspected right ventricular wall MI, consider giving an IV fluid bolus to maintain a systolic blood pressure above 100 mmHg.

** See the thrombolytic criteria check sheet on the following page.

Prehospital Checklist for Inclusion/Exclusion Criteria for Thrombolytic Therapy

These are the questions prehospital personnel should ask (time permitting) the patient who is experiencing chest pain and/or if an AMI is suspected to help determine the patient's eligibility for thrombolytic therapy.

Indications for Thrombolytic Therapy:

EKG: ST segment elevation of at least 1 mm in two contiguous precordial leads, two inferior leads, or two lateral leads.

Symptoms suspicious of acute myocardial infarction of less than 6 hours in duration or stuttering chest pain, with the most extreme episode prompting the patient to seek medical attention beginning within the past 6 hours.

Does the patient have a history of any of the following?

Exclusions	YES	NO
Absolute Contraindication		
Previous hemorrhage stroke at any time	_____	_____
Other history of strokes or cardiovascular events within 1 year	_____	_____
Known intracranial neoplasm (tumor/mass)	_____	_____
Active internal bleeding (except menses)	_____	_____
Suspected aortic dissection	_____	_____
Cautions: Relative Contraindications		
Severe uncontrolled hypertension at presentation (BP >180/110)	_____	_____
Other intracerebral pathology	_____	_____

Current use of anticoagulants
(INR greater than 2–3) _____ _____

Known bleeding diathesis (bleeding
disorders) _____ _____

Recent trauma (past 2–4 weeks),
including head trauma _____ _____

Prolonged (greater than 10 min.)
and/or potentially traumatic CPR _____ _____

Recent major surgery (less than 3 weeks) _____ _____

Noncompressible vascular punctures _____ _____

Recent (within the last 2–4 weeks)
internal bleeding _____ _____

For streptokinase/anistreplase:

Prior exposure (especially in previous
2 years) _____ _____

Prior allergic reaction to
streptokinase _____ _____

Possibility of pregnancy/pregnant _____ _____

Active peptic ulcer _____ _____

Suggested Prehospital Treatment for Ventricular Fibrillation (VF) and Pulseless Ventricular Tachycardia (PVT)

Assess the patient
Establish an airway and ventilate
Suction PRN
High flow oxygen via a BVM
Check for a pulse

|

With the "quick look" paddles, verify the rhythm as VF or PVT
With conductive medium defibrillate 200 J - check rhythm
Defibrillate 300 J - check rhythm
Defibrillate 360 J - check rhythm and pulse
Start CPR if no pulse

|

Intubate the patient and verify the tube placement,
establish an IV, apply the limb leads

|

Give epinephrine 1:10,000 1 mg IVP followed by a 20 ml NS flush
or 2 mg ETT whichever comes first, the IV or ETT

|

While circulating the epinephrine, check for a pulse with CPR,
check breath sounds, draw up 1.5 mg/Kg lidocaine

|

Defibrillate at 360 J within 30-60 seconds of administration of the
epinephrine
check the rhythm and pulse, continue CPR
Give the lidocaine IVP followed by a 20 ml NS flush or ETT

|

While circulating the lidocaine, check for a pulse with CPR, check breath sounds, draw up 1 mg 1:10,000 epinephrine

|

Defibrillate at 360 J within 30-60 seconds of administration of the lidocaine
Check the rhythm and pulse, continue CPR
Give the epinephrine IVP followed by a 20 ml NS flush or ETT

|

While circulating the epinephrine, Check for a pulse with CPR, check breath sounds, draw up 1.5 mg/Kg lidocaine

|

Defibrillate at 360 J within 30-60 seconds of administration of the epinephrine
Check the rhythm and pulse, continue CPR
Give the lidocaine IVP followed by a 20 ml NS flush or ETT

|

While circulating the lidocaine, check for a pulse with CPR, check breath sounds, draw up 1 mg 1:10,000 epinephrine

|

Defibrillate at 360 J within 30-60 seconds of administration of the lidocaine
Check the rhythm and pulse, continue CPR
Give the epinephrine IVP followed by a 20 ml NS flush or ETT

|

While circulating the epinephrine, check for a pulse with CPR, check breath sounds, draw up bretylium 5 mg/Kg

|

Defibrillate at 360 J within 30-60 seconds of administration of the
epinephrine
Check the rhythm and pulse, continue CPR
Give the bretylium IVP followed by a 20 ml NS flush

|

While circulating the bretylium, check for a pulse with CPR,
check breath sounds, draw up 1 mg 1:10,000 epinephrine

|

Defibrillate at 360 J within 30-60 seconds of administration of the
bretylium
Check the rhythm and pulse, continue CPR
Give the epinephrine IVP followed by a 20 ml NS flush or ETT

|

While circulating the epinephrine, check for a pulse with CPR,
check breath sounds, draw up bretylium 10 mg/Kg

|

Defibrillate at 360 J within 30-60 seconds of administration of the
epinephrine
Check the rhythm and pulse, continue CPR
Give the bretylium IVP followed by a 20 ml NS flush

|

Repeat the bretylium 10 mg/Kg IVP q 5 min up to 35 mg/Kg while
repeating 1 mg epinephrine doses in between
continuing CPR and defibrillating at 360 J after every
medication dose given

|

Consider sodium bicarbonate 1 mEq/Kg IVP
Consider magnesium sulfate 1-2 grams IVP
Consider procainamide 30 mg/minute up to 17 mg/Kg

Suggested Prehospital Treatment for Wide QRS Complex Tachycardia (Ventricular Tachycardia)

Assess the patient
Establish an airway and administer oxygen
Check for a pulse
Obtain a set of vital signs, pulse oximetry
Obtain a patient history

|

Attach the limb leads and determine the underlying rhythm

|

Establish an IV

|

Determine if the patient is stable or unstable with signs and/or symptoms of chest pain, SOB, a decreased level of consciousness, hypotension, pulmonary edema, or possible AMI

|

If the patient is conscious, consider a trial dose of medication prior to cardioversion

|

Give lidocaine 1.5 mg/Kg IVP repeating at 0.75 mg/Kg every 5-10 minutes up to 3 mg/Kg

Give procainamide at 20 mg/minute by mixing 1 gram (10 ml) in 40 ml NS to equal 20 mg/ml concentration. Using a 60 gtt/ml IV set up, infuse at 60 gtts/min up to 17 mg/Kg or until hypotension occurs or the rhythm is suppressed

|

Give a bretylium infusion by mixing 5-10 mg/Kg into 50 ml NS and infusing in over 8-10 minutes

If the rhythm is a wide complex tachycardia of an unknown origin (VT vs SVT with aberrancy), give 6 mg adenosine rapid IV push. 12 mg adenosine may be given rapid IV push in 1-2 minutes, and repeated once.

If patient is unconscious with a pulse and has a heart rate over 150 beats per minute, immediately cardiovert at the appropriate energy level while performing pulse checks in between each shock.

|

100 J
200 J
300 J
360 J

If conversion occurs, consider lidocaine suppressive therapy

|

If no conversion occurs, consider lidocaine in between 360 J shocks

Suggested Prehospital Treatment for Ventricular Ectopy and Acute Suppressive Therapy

Assess the patient
Establish an airway
Administer oxygen at 4 L/minute by nasal cannula
Check for a pulse
Obtain a set of vital signs, pulse oximetry
Obtain a patient history

|

Attach the limb leads and determine the underlying rhythm

|

Establish an IV

|

Determine if the patient is stable or unstable with signs and/or symptoms of chest pain, SOB, a decreased level of consciousness, hypotension, pulmonary edema, or possible AMI

|

Suppressive therapy for PVC's is indicated in the symptomatic patient when the PVC's are coupled or paired, multifocal, appear as R on T phenomenon, or as runs of 3 or more PVC's

|

Rule out any treatable causes such as hypoxia, cardiac stimulants

|

Give lidocaine 1.5 mg/Kg IV push

|

If the ectopy is not suppressed, repeat the lidocaine at 0.75 mg/Kg every 3-5 minutes, until the ectopy has been controlled, or up to 3 mg/Kg has been given

|

Once the ectopy has resolved, maintain therapeutic levels by mixing 1 gram of lidocaine into 250 ml NS or 2 grams into 500 ml NS to equal 4 mg/ml and infuse it using the following: *

|

After giving lidocaine 1.5 mg/Kg IV, start the infusion at 2 mg/min (30 gtts/minute)

After giving lidocaine 2.25 mg/Kg IV, start the infusion at 3 mg/min (45 gtts/minute)

After giving lidocaine 3 mg/Kg IV, start the infusion at 4 mg/min (60 gtts/minute)

|

Obtain a 12 lead EKG

* **The drip rate should be cut in half for patients over the age of 70 or those patients with known hepatic disease.**

Suggested Prehosptial Treatment for Narrow QRS Complex Tachycardia (Supraventricular Tachycardia)

Assess the patient, check for a pulse
Establish an airway and administer oxygen
Obtain a set of vital signs, pulse oximetry
Obtain a patient history

Attach the limb leads and determine the underlying rhythm

Establish an IV

Determine if the patient is stable or unstable with signs and/or symptoms of chest pain, SOB, a decreased level of consciousness, hypotension, pulmonary edema, or possible AMI

If the patient is conscious, consider a trial dose of medication for the appropriate rhythm prior to cardioversion	If the patient is unconscious with pulse and has a heart rate over 150 beats per minute

With atrial fibrillation or atrial flutter with a rapid ventricular response and the patient is not hypotensive	With atrial tachycardia or junctional tachycardia try vagal maneuvers	With atrial fibrillation, atrial flutter, atrial tachycardia or junctional tachycardia, immediately cardiovert using settings of:
Give verapamil 2.5 to 5 mg IV slow push given over 2 minutes repeated in 15-20 minutes at 5-10 mg IV slow push, monitoring the patient's blood pressure	Adenosine 6 mg rapid IVP Repeat at 12 mg rapid IVP X 2 every 1-2 minutes	50 J 100 J 200 J 300 J 360 J

If there is no conversion and the patient is not hypotensive, give 2.5 to 5 mg verapamil IV slow push over 2 minutes, repeated in 15-20 minutes at 5-10 mg IV slow push, monitoring the patient's blood pressure

Suggested Prehospital Treatment for Pulseless Electrical Activity (PEA)

(A rhythm is present where a pulse is expected to be found, but is not)

Including:

1. Bradyasystolic rhythms - agonal rhythms with slow, irregular wide QRS complexes.
2. Electromechanical dissociation (EMD) - organized electrical activity on the monitor but no heart muscle contraction (e.g., NSR with no pulse).
3. Idioventricular rhythms, including those that appear after defibrillation.
4. Ventricular escape rhythms.

Assess the patient
Establish an airway
Suction PRN
High flow oxygen via BVM
Check for a pulse

|

With the "quick look" paddles, verify the rhythm as PEA
Start CPR if there is no pulse

|

Intubate patient and verify the tube placement,
establish an IV, apply the limb leads

|

Consider the possible causes and treat if found (treatment):
Hypovolemia is the most common cause (volume infusion)
Acidosis (consider sodium bicarbonate at 1 mEg/Kg)
Cardiac tamponade (pericardiocentesis)
Drug overdoses such as tricyclics, digitalis, beta blockers,
narcotics, calcium channel blockers ("STONED" therapy *)
Hyperkalemia (sodium bicarbonate 1 mEg/Kg)
Hypothermia (see the adult hypothermia treatment protocol p. 62)
Hypoxia (oxygenation/ventilation)

Pulmonary embolism (rapid transport)
Massive AMI (see Chest Pain /AMI treatment p.xx)
Tension pneumothorax (needle decompression)

|

If unsure of cause or cause cannot be found
Give epinephrine 1:10,000 1 mg IVP, repeat every 3-5 minutes

|

If the rhythm is bradycardic
Give atropine 1 mg IVP every 3 minutes up to 3 mg

* "STONED" therapy: Sodium Bicarbonate, Thiamine, Oxygen, Narcan, Even D50

Suggested Prehospital Treatment for Adult Hypothermia

Assess the patient
Establish an airway
Check for a pulse
Administer oxygen (warmed, if possible)
Obtain a set of vital signs, pulse oximetry (if possible)
Obtain a patient history

|

Remove all wet clothing, protect against additional heat loss,
maintain the patient in a supine position and minimize rough
handling and movement during treatment and transport

|

Attach the limb leads and determine the underlying rhythm

|

Establish an IV using warm normal saline

|

Perform a physical exam

A Patient with a Pulse and/or an Organized Cardiac Rhythm

If the patient has a pulse and is still breathing, or there is
no palpable pulse but an organized cardiac rhythm on the
monitor and some respiratory effort; maintain a clear airway,
administer warm humidified oxygen by mask or BVM, and
gently transport the patient to an appropriate medical facility.

OR

A Patient with No Pulse and is in V-Tach or V-Fib

If the patient is pulseless and apneic, and the monitor shows
ventricular tachycardia or ventricular fibrillation

|

Start CPR

|

Defibrillate a total of 3 times at: 200 J, 300 J, 360 J
Check for a pulse and rhythm change

|

Continue CPR if no conversion has occurred

|

Carefully intubate the patient
and verify the tube placement

|

Gently transport the patient to an appropriate medical facility

|

Do not administer any medications unless directed
by medical control

Suggested Prehospital Treatment for Hypotension, Shock, and Acute Pulmonary Edema

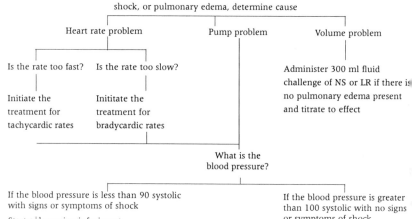

Assess the patient
Establish an airway and administer oxygen
Check for a pulse
Obtain a set of vital signs, pulse oximetry
Obtain a patient history

Attach the limb leads and determine the underlying rhythm

Establish an IV

Perform physical exam

If there is a problem with hypotension, shock, or pulmonary edema, determine cause

Heart rate problem | **Pump problem** | **Volume problem**

Is the rate too fast?   Is the rate too slow?

Initiate the treatment for tachycardic rates

Inititate the treatment for bradycardic rates

Administer 300 ml fluid challenge of NS or LR if there is no pulmonary edema present and titrate to effect

What is the blood pressure?

If the blood pressure is less than 90 systolic with signs or symptoms of shock

Start a dopamine infusion at 2-20mcg/Kg/minute

If the blood pressure is greater than 100 systolic with no signs or symptoms of shock

Start a nitroglycerin infusion at 10-20 mcg/minute

If pulmonary edema exists or continues

Consider lasix 0.5 - 1 mg/Kg slow IVP
Consider morphine 1-3 mg slow IVP
Consider nitroglycerin 0.3-0.4 mg SL
Consider intubation
Consider positive pressure ventilation

Suggested Prehospital Treatment for Asystole

Assess the patient
Establish an airway
Suction PRN
High flow oxygen via BVM
Check for a pulse

|

With the "quick look" paddles, verify the rhythm as asystole
Reconfirm asystole by moving the left leg paddle
up to the left chest paddle position (Lead I)

|

Start CPR if no pulse

|

Intubate the patient and verify the tube placement,
establish an IV, apply the limb leads

|

Consider the possible causes and treat if found (treatment):
Hypothermia (see the adult hypothermia treatment protocol p. 62)
Acidosis (consider sodium bicarbonate at 1 mEg/Kg)
Drug overdose (specific treatments, "STONED" therapy*)
Hypoxia (oxygenation/ventilation)

|

If unsure of cause or no cause found
Consider transcutaneous pacing ** if a witnessed arrest ***

|

Give epinephrine 1:10,000 1 mg IVP,
repeating every 3-5 minutes

|

Give atropine sulfate 1 mg IVP every 3-5 minutes
up to 3 mg or 0.04 mg/Kg

|

Circulate the drugs well with CPR,
Check pulses with CPR, check breath sounds

|

After three doses of epinephrine and atropine sulfate
Consider terminating the arrest

* "STONED" Therapy: Sodium Bicarbonate, Thiamine, Oxygen, Narcan, Even D50.

** If transcutaneous pacing is used for asystole, set the pacer at 200 milliamps at a rate of 100 BPM.

*** Witness arrest: A visual change on the monitor from a rhythm with electrical activity to asystole.

Suggested Prehospital Treatment for Bradycardic Rhythms

Assess the patient
Establish an airway
Check for a pulse
Administer oxygen
Obtain a set of vital signs, pulse oximetry
Obtain a patient history
|

Attach the limb leads and determine the underlying rhythm
|

Establish an IV
|

Perform a physical exam
|

Determine if the patient is stable or unstable with signs and/or symptoms of chest pain, SOB, a decreased level of consciousness, hypotension, pulmonary edema, or possible AMI
|

Determine if the rate is less than 60 BPM or if a relative bradycardia with a rate 60-65 is present (producing an unstable patient)

If the bradycardia produces no signs or symptoms, monitor only, unless

If the bradycardia is producing signs or symptoms

If the rhythm is a 2nd degree Mobitz Type II HB or 3rd degree HB

Attach the TCP * and prepare to pace the patient using sedation or analgesia as needed.**

Give 0.5-1.0 mg of atropine IVP repeating at 1.0 mg every 3-5 minutes up to 3 mg while attaching a transcutaneous pacer * (TCP), if available. If atropine is refractory and a TCP is unavailable, consider a dopamine infusion at 5-20 mcg/Kg/minute, or epinephrine infusion at 2-10 mcg/Kg/minute.

* If TCP is used for bradycardia, set the pacer at 80 BPM and start it at 20 milliamps, increasing by 20 milliamps until mechanical capture (a pulse) is obtained.

** When pacing a conscious patient, consider using Versed or Valium for sedation.

Emergency Cardiac Pacing

Anterior-Anterior Electrode Placement

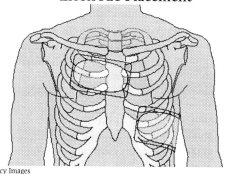

LifeART Emergency Images
Copyright © 1994 TechPool Studios Corp. USA

Anterior-Anterior

Place one pad on the right anterior chest wall below the clavicle and to the right of the sternum. Place the other pad on the lower left chest wall above the lowest rib at the anterior axillary line.

Anterior-Posterior

Place one pad on the right anterior chest wall below the clavicle and to the right of the sternum. Place the other pad on the back in between the spine and the left scapula below the lower angle of the left scapula.

Bradycardia: Set the rate between 60-80 BPM and the amperage at 20 mA, increase the mA by 20 until electrical capture (QRS following pacer spikes) is noted on EKG. Increase mA by 5–20 mA until mechanical capture (a pulse) is noted.

Asystole: Set the rate between 80-100 BPM and the amperage at 200 mA and look for both electrical and mechanical capture.

Obstetrics and Neonatal

Fundal Height Chart

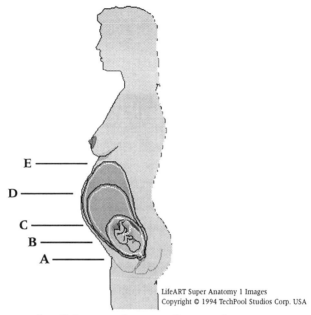

LifeART Super Anatomy 1 Images
Copyright © 1994 TechPool Studios Corp. USA

Relative Levels of the Uterine Fundus During Pregnancy
(as measured from the level of the pubis (A) to the top of the uterus)

	Location	Length of Pregnancy	Trimester
B	Halfway between pubis and umbilicus	12 weeks	1st
C	Level of umbilicus	20–22 weeks	2nd
D	Halfway between umbilicus and xiphoid	28 weeks	2nd
E	Below xiphoid	40 weeks	3rd

Suggested Prehospital Treatment for Neonatal Resuscitation

Pre-delivery Considerations

Obtain a patient history (if possible) prior to delivery

|

High-risk maternal history that may increase the potential for delivery of a depressed newborn include:

Mother is older than 35 or younger than 16 years of age

No prenatal care

Multiple babies are present

History of diabetes, drug abuse, pre-eclampsia, hypertension, abruptioplacenta, placenta previa or complications with previous births

Pre-term delivery

History or presence of meconium staining

Use of narcotics/opiates within the last four hours

|

Additional field delivery considerations (imminent delivery):

Contractions are less than 2 to 3 minutes apart

Mother has an uncontrolled urge to push

Infant is crowning

Second or more delivery for the mother and she says she is going to deliver at any time

Delivery of a Depressed or Asphyxiated Newborn

Prepare for the delivery of the newborn

|

Manage breach deliveries and prolapsed cord appropriately

|

Assist in the delivery

Delivery

At the delivery of the newborn head, observe for the **umbilical cord** around the infant's neck.

Look for the presence of **meconium staining** in the amniotic fluid or on the infant's skin.
If there is no meconium noted, use a regular bulb syringe and suction the mouth, then nose of the newborn as the head delivers.

After the delivery of the infant, dry and position the infant on the back with the shoulders elevated about 1 inch to maintain neutral head alignment.
Assure a patent airway.

Suction the airway as needed.

Specific Treatments

If the umbilical cord is around the baby's neck, gently loosen the cord and slide it over the baby's head.

If **meconium staining** is noted, it is important to suction the newborn **before** the baby is delivered and **before** its first breath. This is best done by direct intubation as the head is delivered. Once the ET tube is placed, a portable suction unit can be used to suction the end of the ET tube as the tube is withdrawn.

Repeat as needed, up to 3 times before ventilating with a BVM. The suction pressure should be limited to -100 mmHg and no more.

Suctioning should be limited to 3-5 seconds with hyperoxygenation before and after. Remember that deep oral suctioning can cause bradycardia.

Delivery

Specific Treatments

Stimulate the infant by gently flicking the feet or rubbing the back or head. Keep the infant warm and dry. Immediately assess the infant's color, muscle activity, heart rate, respiratory status, and reflexes. Mentally assign an **APGAR** score at 1 and 5 minutes.

See the **APGAR** scoring chart.

If the infant is breathing on its own but appears dusky in color and has weak muscle tone, administer **oxygen.**

100% **oxygen** can be given by mask or by the blow by method using 10 to 12 liters per minute.

If the infant is not breathing or their respirations do not improve with oxygen, immediately begin positive pressure **ventilation** with a BVM.

Ventilations should be done with a BVM attached to 100% oxygen delivered at a rate of 40 to 60 breaths per minute.
Be careful when ventilating newborns. They require smaller tidal volumes than older children, but slightly more ventilation pressure. Continuously assess for breath sounds and look for chest rise.

Check the infant's heart rate and pulse by palpating the base of the umbilical cord, or the femoral or brachial artery. The heart rate should greater than 100 BPM. If the heart rate is less than 100 BPM, begin positive pressure ventilation with a BVM and consider **intubation** if needed.

Intubation should be done if there are problems using a BVM, or prolonged use; presence of thick meconium in the airway; or the baby has meconium staining and is born "floppy." Reassess the ETT tube to assure the tube is still properly placed and has not become obstructed. Avoid increased ventilation pressures. Monitor for the presence of a pneumothorax and/or gastric distention.

Delivery

If the heart rate is less than 60 BPM or between 60 and 80 BPM and not improving with positive pressure ventilation, begin **CPR**.

If the heart rate remains at 80 BPM or less despite CPR, intubation, and oxygenation, establish **IV** access as quickly and safely as possible using normal saline solution.

Give 0.1-0.3 ml/Kg (0.01-0.03 mg/Kg) of 1:10,000 epinephrine IV, IO or 0.1 every 3-5 minutes until the heart rate improves above 100 ml/Kg of 1:1,000 epinephrine **ETT** without CPR.

Consider giving Narcan 0.1 mg/Kg IV, IO, ETT if the mother has received any narcotics in the previous 4 hours.

Consider checking a **glucose** level and if needed, giving D10 IV or IO.

Specific Treatments

CPR should be done at a rate of 12 compressions a minute at a depth of 1/2 to 3/4 inches or until a strong pulse is palpated.

IV access can be obtained by an IV route (hands, feet, scalp) IO or if trained, the umbilical vein.

ETT doses should be diluted in 3-5 ml of normal saline.

Blood **glucose** level in a newborn should be above 40 mg/dl.

The APGAR Score

Sign	0	1	2
Appearance (Skin color)	Blue, pale	Body pink, extremities blue	Completely pink
Pulse Rate (Heart rate)	Absent	Below 100	Above 100
Grimace (Irritability)	No response	Grimaces	Cries
Activity (Muscle tone)	Limp	Some flexion of extremities	Active motion
Respiratory (Effort)	Absent	Slow and irregular	Strong cry

Score 1 Minute: _____ **Score 5 Minutes:** _____ **Score 10 Minutes:** _____

Pediatrics

Pediatric Formulas
(Children 10 years old and under)

Respiration and Pulse:

By knowing the average respiration rate of a child, the normal heart rate can be "ballparked" by multiplying the respiratory rate by 5. Notice the adolescent respiratory rate of 15 is just about the same as the adult. Add 5 to each age group and it becomes fairly easy to remember. This should get you through your initial assessment.

STAGE	Age	Respiration	(Times 5) =	Pulse
Newborn	0-1	30	(x 5)	150
Preschool	1-5	25	(x 5)	125
School age	5-8	20	(x 5)	100
Adolescent	8-10	15	(x 5)	75

Kilogram Weight: 2 (age) + 8 = Kilograms (Kg)

Example: 2 (3 y/o) + 8 = 14 Kg (31 lbs)

ET Tube Size: $\dfrac{Age\ (yrs.) + 16}{4}$ **OR** $\dfrac{Age\ (yrs.)\ (+ 4\ )}{4}$

Example:

$\dfrac{3\ y/o + 16}{4} = 4.75$ or $\dfrac{3\ y/o\ (+ 4\ )}{4} = 4.75$

5.0 I.D.   or 5.0 I.D.

Blood Volume: 80 mL/Kg

Blood Pressure: 2 (age) + 80 = systolic

2/3 systolic = diastolic

Temperatures: Normal (oral) - 98.6

Rectal - one degree higher than oral

Axillary - one degree lower than oral

Fluid Administration: 20 milliliters x kilogram weight = fluid bolus to be given

Electrical Energy: Defibrillation: 2 joules/Kg repeat at 4 joules/Kg

Cardioversion: 0.5 joules/Kg repeat at 1 joules/Kg

Suggested Prehospital Treatment for Pediatric Bradycardic Rhythms

Assess the patient

Establish an airway and administer oxygen

Check for a pulse

Obtain a set of vital signs, pulse oximetry

Obtain a patient history

|

Attach the limb leads and determine the underlying rhythm

|

Perform a physical exam

|

Determine if the patient is stable or unstable with signs and/or symptoms of cardiopulmonary compromise including respiratory difficulty or arrest, poor peripheral perfusion and/or hypotension

|

Stable Condition

Observe and monitor for decompensation into an unstable condition. Support the patient's airway and breathing status, transport to a medical facility.

Unstable Condition

Ventilate with a BVM and 100% oxygen. Consider intubation if there is difficulty maintaining an airway with the BVM. If the heart rate drops below 60 (child) or 80 (infant) despite ventilatory support, begin CPR at a rate of 100 compressions a minute.

|

Establish an IV or IO access.
Give epinephrine 1:10,000
0.1 ml/Kg (0.01 mg/Kg) IV/IO or
1:1,000 at 0.1 ml/Kg ETT
every 3 to 5 minutes.

|

Consider atropine 0.02 mg/Kg
IV, IO. ETT: 0.04-0.06 mg/Kg
Minimum dose all ages (0.1 mg)
Children less than 5 years old:
Maximum single dose is 0.5 mg
Maximum total dose is 1.0 mg
Children over 5 years old:
Maximum single dose is 1.0 mg
Maximum total dose is 2.0 mg

|

Consider sodium bicarbonate
1 mEq/Kg IV/IO.

Suggested Prehospital Treatment for Pediatric Asystole/Arrest

Assess the patient
Establish an airway
Suction PRN
High flow oxygen via BVM
Check for a pulse

|

With the "quick look" paddles, verify the rhythm as asystole
Reconfirm asystole by moving the left leg paddle
up to the left chest paddle position (Lead I)

|

Start CPR if no pulse

|

Intubate the patient and verify the tube placement,
Establish an IV or IO, apply the limb leads

|

Consider the possible causes and treat if found (treatment):
Acidosis (insure proper ventilation/oxygenation
then consider sodium bicarbonate: 1 mEq/Kg IV or IO)
Cardiac tamponade (rapid transport)
Hypoxia (oxygenation/ventilation)
Hypothermia (see the pediatric hypothermia
treatment protocol)
Hypovolemia (fluid volume replacement)
Tension pneumothorax (needle decompression)

|

Give epinephrine 1:10,000 IV, IO: 0.1 ml/Kg (0.01mg/Kg)
or

1:1,000 ETT: 0.1 ml/Kg (0.1 mg/Kg)

|

All repeat doses of epinephrine should be
at 0.1 ml/Kg (0.1 mg/Kg) IV, IO or ETT of 1:1,000
every 3 to 5 minutes

|

Circulate the drugs well with CPR,
check pulses with CPR, check breath sounds,
consider doing a glucometer for hypoglycemia

Suggested Prehospital Treatment for Pediatric Tachycardic Rhythms

Assess the patient

Establish an airway and administer oxygen

Check for a pulse

Obtain a set of vital signs, pulse oximetry

Obtain a patient history

|

Attach the limb leads and determine the underlying rhythm by reviewing the patient's history, performing a physical exam, looking at the heart rate and width of the QRS, and then comparing the information to the chart below

|

Determine if the patient is stable or unstable

Stable	**Unstable**
If the patient is stable, consider an IV, monitor the patient, and	If the patient is unstable presenting with signs and/or symptoms of hypotension,
transport them to an appropriate medical facility.	cardiopulmonary compromise, or any other signs of poor perfusion, begin to assist the patient by:
	Establishing an IV or IO, and consider the treatment of choice based on the underlying rhythm that's determined.

Sinus Tachycardia	SVT	Ventricular Tachycardia
|	|	|

Heart Rate

Less than 220 - infant	Greater than 220 - infant	Greater than 220 - infant
Less than 180 - child	Greater than 180 - child	Greater than 180 - child

QRS Width

The QRS is narrow	The QRS is narrow	The QRS is wide

History

May be history of pain, fever, trauma; volume loss from diarrhea, vomiting, sepsis or dehydration	Nonspecific history of irritability, poor feeding, pallor, or tachypnea	May have a specific history of congenital heart disease, or some other cardiac history.
		There may be no specific history other than pallor or irritability.

Treatment

Oxygen/ventilation. Treat the underlying cause. For volume depletion give 20 ml/Kg NS IV, IO and repeat as needed based on the heart rate, peripheral pulses, muscle tone and blood pressure. If blood pressure support is further needed, consider a dopamine or epinephrine infusion. (See the Pediatric Dopamine and Epinephrine Infusion Charts)	Oxygen/ventilation Consider adenosine 0.1 mg/Kg (Max 6 mg) IV, IO rapid push. Repeat at 0.2 mg/Kg (Max 12 mg). Cardiovert at 0.5 J/Kg and repeat at 1.0 J/Kg.	Oxygen/ventilation Cardiovert at 0.5 J/Kg and repeat at 1.0 J/Kg. Consider lidocaine IV, IO 1 mg/Kg q 10-15 min. or bretylium IV, IO 5 mg/Kg up to 35 mg/Kg. (See the Pediatric Lidocaine Infusion Chart)
		Note: Ventricular arrhythmias in infants and children are very rare.

Suggested Prehospital Treatment for Pediatric Ventricular Fibrillation (VF) or Pulseless Ventricular Tachycardia (PVT)

Assess the patient

Establish an airway and ventilate

Suction PRN

High flow oxygen via a BVM

Check for a pulse

|

With the "quick look" paddles, verify the rhythm as VF or PVT

With conductive medium defibrillate at 2 J/Kg
- check the rhythm

Defibrillate at 4 J/Kg - check the rhythm

Defibrillate at 4 J/Kg - check the rhythm and pulse

Start CPR if no pulse

|

Intubate the patient and verify tube the placement,
establish an IV or IO, apply the limb leads

|

Give epinephrine 1:10,000 0.1 ml/Kg (0.01 mg/Kg) IV, IO
or 0.1 ml/Kg of 1:1,000 ETT—whichever comes first,
the IV/IO or ETT

|

While circulating the epinephrine, check for a pulse with CPR,
check breath sounds, draw up 1 mg/Kg lidocaine

|

Defibrillate at 4 J/Kg within 30-60 seconds of administration of the epinephrine

Check the rhythm and pulse, continue CPR

Give the lidocaine IVP or IO followed by a small NS flush

|

While circulating the lidocaine, check for a pulse with CPR, check breath sounds, draw up 0.1 ml/Kg 1:1,000 epinephrine

|

Defibrillate at 4 J/Kg within 30-60 seconds of administration of the lidocaine

Check the rhythm and pulse, continue CPR

Give the epinephrine IVP or IO followed by a small NS flush

|

While circulating the epinephrine, check for a pulse with CPR, check breath sounds, draw up 1 mg/Kg lidocaine

|

Defibrillate at 4 J/Kg within 30-60 seconds of administration of the epinephrine

Check the rhythm and pulse, continue CPR

Give the lidocaine IVP or IO followed by a small NS flush

|

While circulating the lidocaine, check for a pulse with CPR, check breath sounds, draw up 0.1 ml/Kg 1:1,000 epinephrine

|

Defibrillate at 4 J/Kg within 30-60 seconds of administration of the lidocaine

Check the rhythm and pulse, continue CPR

Give the epinephrine IVP or IO followed by a small NS flush

|

While circulating the epinephrine, check for a pulse with CPR, check breath sounds, draw up bretylium 5 mg/Kg

|

Consider sodium bicarbonate 1 mEq/Kg IVP

|

Defibrillate at 4 J/Kg within 30-60 seconds of administration of the epinephrine

Check the rhythm and pulse, continue CPR

Give the bretylium IVP or IO followed by a small NS flush

|

While circulating the bretylium, check for a pulse with CPR, check breath sounds, draw up 0.1 ml/Kg 1:1,000 epinephrine

|

Defibrillate at 4 J/Kg within 30-60 seconds of administration of the bretylium

Check the rhythm and pulse, continue CPR

Give the epinephrine IVP or IO followed by a small NS flush

|

While circulating the epinephrine, check for a pulse with CPR, check breath sounds, draw up bretylium 10 mg/Kg

|

Defibrillate at 4 J/Kg within 30-60 seconds of administration of the epinephrine

Check rhythm and pulse, continue CPR

Give the bretylium IVP or IO followed by a small NS flush

|

Repeat bretylium 10 mg/Kg IVP every 5 minutes up to
35 mg/Kg while repeating 0.1 ml/Kg 1:1,000 epinephrine
doses in between continuing CPR and defibrillating at
4 J/Kg in between doses

Suggested Prehospital Treatment for Pediatric Hypothermia

Assess the patient

Establish an airway

Check for a pulse

Administer oxygen (warmed, if possible)

Obtain a set of vital signs, pulse oximetry (if possible)

Obtain a patient history

|

Remove all wet clothing, protect against additional heat loss, maintain the patient in a supine position and minimize rough handling and movement during treatment and transport

|

Attach the limb leads and determine the underlying rhythm

|

Perform a physical exam

A Patient with a Pulse and/or an Organized Cardiac Rhythm

If the patient has both a pulse and respirations, or if the patient has respiratory effort with an organized cardiac rhythm on the monitor but no palpable pulse; maintain a clear airway and administer oxygen by mask, warm the patient with blankets and wrapped hot packs placed around the groin, neck, and armpits; consider an IV if warm fluids are available, and gently transport the patient to an appropriate medical facility

OR

A Patient with No Pulse and is in V-Tach or V-Fib

If the patient is pulseless and apneic, and the monitor shows
ventricular tachycardia or ventricular fibrillation

|

Start CPR

|

Defibrillate a total of 3 times at: 2 J/Kg, 4 J/Kg, 4 J/Kg

Check for a pulse and rhythm change

|

Continue CPR if no conversion occurred

|

Carefully intubate the patient and verify the tube placement

|

Consider an IV or IO

|

Gently transport the patient to an appropriate medical facility

|

Do not administer any medications unless directed

Pediatric Trauma Scale

Severity	+2	+1	-1
Weight	> 44 lbs (> 20 kg)	22 to 44 lbs (10-20 kg)	< 22 lbs (< 10 kg)
Airway	Normal	Oral or nasal airway	Invasive: intubation cricothyrotomy
Blood pressure and/or pulses	> 90 mmHg or radial pulse only	50 to 90 mmHg Femoral pulse only	< 50 mmHg or absent pulse
Level of consciousness	Awake Alert	Obtunded, any loss of consciousness; verbal or painful response only	Comatose Unresponsive
Open wounds	None	Minor	Major or penetrating
Fractures	None	Single, simple	Open or multiple

Pediatric Coma Scale

Eye Opening

		SCORE	Initial (Time)	In Route (Time)
≥ 1 Year	**< 1 Year**			
Spontaneously	Spontaneously	4	4	
To verbal command	To shout	3	3	
To pain	To pain	2	2	
No response	No response	1	1	

Best Motor Responses

≥ 1 Year	**< 1 Year**			
Obeys	Spontaneously	6	6	
Localizes pain	Localizes pain	5	5	
Flexion-withdrawal	Flexion-withdrawal	4	4	
Flexion-abnormal (decorticate rigidity)	Flexion-abnormal (decorticate rigidity)	3	3	
Extension (decerebrate rigidity)	Extension (decerebrate rigidity)	2	2	
No response	No response	1	1	

Best Verbal Responses

≥ 5 Years	**2 to 5 Years**	**0 to 23 Months**		
Oriented and converses	Appropriate words/phrases	Smiles and coos appropriately	5	5

> 5 Years	2 to 5 Years	0 to 23 Months	SCORE	Initial (Time)	In Route (Time)
Disoriented and converses	Inappropriate words	Cries and is consolable		4	4
Inappropriate words	Persistent crying and screaming	Persistent and/or inappropriate crying and/or screaming		3	3
Incomprehensible sounds	Grunts	Grunts, agitated, and restless		2	2
No response	No response	No response		1	1

TOTAL = 3 to 15

Neurological

Levels of Consciousness

Assessment and Patient Response   AVPU System

1. Alert and oriented to person, place, and time - (A/O X 3).

2. Alert and oriented to person and place - (A/O X 2).   **ALERT**

3. Alert and oriented to place only - (A/O X 1).

4. Unconscious but responds to simple verbal commands ("open your eyes", "squeeze my hand").   **VERBAL**

5. Unconscious but responds to pain with purposeful movements (localizes the pain).

6. Unconscious but responds to pain with nonpurposeful movements (withdraw from pain with decorticate or decerebrate posturing).   **PAINFUL**

7. Unconscious but gag and corneal reflexes are still present.

8. Unconscious and unresponsive to any stimulus(flaccid).   **UNCONSCIOUS**

Considerations for Altered Levels of Consciousness/Coma

AEIOU - Tips

A	-	Acidosis, Alcohol, Anaphylaxis
E	-	Epilepsy, Electrolytes, Environmental
I	-	Insulin (too much, too little)
O	-	Overdose, Obstruction (airway)
U	-	Uremia
T	-	Trauma, Temperature
I	-	Infections, Injections
P	-	Psychosis, Poisoning
S	-	Strokes

Humane (painless) assessment methods for determining "suspicious" alerted Level of Consciousness.

Arm Drop Test

With the patient supine, lift the patient's arm 12-14 inches above their face and let the arm drop toward their face. Probable unconscious state: The patient's arm falls rapidly hitting the patient's face. "Suspicious" results: the patient's arm falls in a more controlled drop glancing the side of their head or missing their head and face altogether.

Buzzing Bee/Fly Test

(Best done in a room or in the back of your unit.) While at the patient's side state to your partner that there is a bee/fly in the room/unit bothering you. (You or your partner can add sound effects if you want.) After a few minutes of attempting to rid of the pest, take a cotton tip applicator or the cover of a gauze

pad and lightly touch the inside of the patient's nostril.
<u>Probable unconscious state:</u> The patient does nothing.
<u>Suspicious results:</u> The patient attempts to remove the
"bee/fly" from their nose by blowing their nose or wiping their
nose with their hand.

Insulin and Glucometers
Types of Insulin for Injection

	<u>Onset</u>	<u>Duration of Action</u>
Short Acting		
Humalog	5 minutes	2-4 hours
Insulin (regular)	1/2-1 hour	6-8 hours
Combination		
50/50 or 70/30	1/2-1 hour	18-24 hours
Intermediate		
NPH	1-2 hours	18-24 hours
Lente	1-3 hours	18-24 hours
Long Acting		
(UL) Ultralente	6 hours	24-28 hours

Types of Oral Hypoglycemic Medications

Diabeta
(Glyburide)

Glucophage
(Metformin Hydrochloride)

Diabinese
(Chlorpropamide)

Micronase
(Glyburide)

Dymelor
(Acetohexamide)

Orinase
(Tolbutamide)

Glucotrol
(Glipzide)

Precose
(Acarbose)

Glucotrol XL
(Glipzide)

Rezulin
(Troglitazone)

Glynase
(Micronized)

Tolinase
(Tolazamide)

Using a Glucometer

Be sure that the reagent strips are the same code as the code display on the glucometer when it is turned on. The glucometers are calibrated to measure capillary blood only. This means to obtain the most accurate glucose reading you should perform a finger stick to obtain your blood sample, not from an IV start. If you use blood from an IV, the venous glucose reading could be 10% to 20% different than the capillary reading.

Lowest Acceptable Levels
of Normal Blood Glucose

Adult: 80 mg/dl

Child: 60 mg/dl

Neonate: 40 mg/dl

Prehospital Stroke Assessment

Have the patient:	Look for:
Hold both arms out straight in front of them with palms up and close their eyes while listening to your count.	Any arm drifting downward or palm pronating while you count for 10-15 seconds out loud.
Stick out their tongue as straight as possible.	Their tongue moving or pointing toward one corner of their mouth.
Smile and show their teeth with their jaw clinched.	Any drop of either side of their mouth.
Squeeze your wrists with both hands simultaneously as hard as they can.	Any noticeable weakness in grip strength of either hand.
Push and pull their feet (dorsi/plantar flex) against your hands as hard as they can.	Any noticeable weakness in strength of either foot.
Name an object after you tell them what it is (i.e., stethoscope, dictionary) or recite a short sentence (i.e., "Do you know what time it is?").	Abnormal, slurred, garbled or absences of their speech.
Look at your face and then without turning their head, look up, down, left, and right.	Any inability to look in any of these directions or the eyes deviate toward one side with noor little movement.

If any of these findings are present, consider the possibility of a CVA or TIA.

Common Street Names
for Various Medications

DRUG	STREET NAME	SIGNS/SYMPTOMS

1. AMPHETAMINES
("Uppers")

a. Amphetamine	Bennies, Black Beauties, Black Mollies, Bombita Cartwheels, Crossroads, Lid Proppers, Jelly Babies, Peaches, Purple Hearts, Roes, Uppers	**OVERDOSE:** Agitation, combative tachycardia, dilated pupils, possible chest pain, diaphoresis, nausea, vomiting, ischemia
b. Dexedrine	Dexies, Oranges, Footballs	**WITHDRAWAL:**
c. MDEA	Eve	Sleepiness, hard to arouse, increased appetite, muscle cramps, diarrhea
d. Methedrine	Crank, Meth, Speed	
e. MDMA	Adam, Ecstasy, X, XTC	

2. BARBITURATES
("Downers")

a. Phenobarbital (Nembutal)	Barbs, Nemmines, Nimbies, Nolo, Yellow Jackets, Yellows	**OVERDOSE:** Hard to arouse, shallow respirations
b. Amytal	Blue Birds, Blue Devils	**WITHDRAWAL:** Tremors, GI symptoms, agitation, abdominal cramps, anxiety
c. Seconal	Red Birds, Red Devils, F-40's, Mexican Reds, Pinks, Red Lillies, Seccy	
d. Tuinal	Christmas Trees, T-birds, Rainbows	

3. COCAINE

a. Cocaine Powder	"C", Bernice, Bernies Flake, Big Bloke, Carrie, Flake, Dream, Dust, Happy Dust,	**OVERDOSE:** Agitation, hypertension, chest pain (MI), warm skin

DRUG	STREET NAME	SIGNS/SYMPTOMS
	Lady, Nose Candy, Snow, Star Dust, The Leaf, Joy Power, Girl, Smack	**WITHDRAWAL:** Depression, hard to arouse
b. Crack	Rock, Ice	

---

4. HASHISH Hash, Keif	**OVERDOSE:** Same as Marijuana **WITHDRAWAL:** Same as Marijuana

---

5. LYSERGIC ACID

a. Diethylamine (LSD)	Acid, Battery Acid, Big D, Black Sunshine, Blue Acid, Microdot, Domes, Strawberry Field, Sunshine, Purple Haze, Window Pane, Window Glass, Zen, Wedding Bells	**OVERDOSE:** Hallucinations, psychosis, mood swings, aggressive behavior, dilated pupils **WITHDRAWAL:** Depression, mood swings

---

6. MARIJUANA

	Acapulco Gold, Bhang Bush, Charge, Giggle Smoke, Gold, Grass, Hay, Hemp, Herb, Joint, Indian Hay, Doobie, Locoweed, MJ, Mary Jane, Panama Red, Pot, Reefer, Rope, Straw, Tea, Weed	**OVERDOSE:** Tired, paranoid **WITHDRAWAL:** Depression

---

7. OPIOIDS/NARCOTICS

a. Codeine	School Boy	**OVERDOSE:** Hypotension, bradycardia, shallow to absent respirations, pulmonary
b. Heroin	Big Harry, Boy, Dope, Dynamite, Hairy, Horse	

DRUG	STREET NAME	SIGNS/SYMPTOMS
	Smack, Skag, TNT, Joy Power, China White	edema, pinpoint pupils
		WITHDRAWAL:
c. Dilaudid	Lords	Agitation, GI symptoms, shakes, clammy skin, tachycardia, rhinorrhea, hallucinations including auditory, visual, and tactile
d. Fentanyl	China White, Tango and Cash	
e. Methadone	Dolls, Dollies	
f. Morphine	Unkie, Miss Emma, Morph, Emsel, Hard Stuff, Cube Juice	

8. METHAQUALONE
(Quaalude)
Lude, Quary, Sopers, Soapers, 714's

OVERDOSE:

Hallucinations, hypotension, shallow respirations

WITHDRAWAL:
Seizures, GI symptoms, hypertension

9. PEYOTE
(Mescaline)
Bad Seed, Cactus, Moon Mese, Mesc

OVERDOSE:

Same as LSD

WITHDRAWAL:
Seizures, GI symptoms, hypertension. Vomiting is very common when anyone takes peyote.

DRUG	STREET NAME	SIGNS/SYMPTOMS

10. PHENCYCLIDINE
    (PCP)

Angel Dust, Angel Hair, Peace Pill, Hog, Dusted Parsley, Horse Tranquilizer

OVERDOSE:
Violent episodes, paranoia, increased perception of muscle strength, decreased pain response, hypertension

WITHDRAWAL:
Depression, hard to arouse

Antidotes to Common Medications and Drugs

Medication/Drug	Antidote	Suggested Dose
Acetaminophen	N-acetylcysteine (mucomyst)	Initially 140 mg/Kg PO
Anticholinergics (Atropine)	Physostigmine (Antilirium)	Adults: 2 mg slow IV Pediatrics: 0.5 mg slow IV
Benzodiazepines (Valium) (Versed)	Flumazenil (Romazicon) (Mazicon)	0.2 mg IV over 30 seconds repeated at 0.5 mg up to a total dose of 3 mg
Sympatholytics (Beta Blockers)	Glucagon	1 mg slow IV (use D5W IV solution only, no saline solution)
Calcium Channel Blockers (Verapamil)	Calcium chloride	500-200 mg (5-20 ml) slow IV
Ingested Poisons	Activated charcoal	15-30 ml mixed in water
Cyanide	Amyl nitrate pearls	Inhale for 30 seconds times 2 over 1 minute
	Sodium Nitrate	Adult: 10 ml (300 mg) IV over 20 minutes Pediatric: 0.2 ml/Kg IV up to 10 ml over 20 minutes
	Sodium thiosulfate	Adult: 50 ml (12.5 grams) IV over 20 minute. Pediatric: 1 ml/Kg IV over 20 minutes
Organophosphates (Cholesterase Inhibitors)	Atropine	Adult: 2 mg IV repeated until respirations improve Pediatric: 0.05 mg/Kg IV until respirations improve

Medication/Drug	Antidote	Suggested Dose
Narcotics (Opioids)	Narcan (Naloxone)	Adult: 2 mg IV, may repeat X 2 up to 10 mg Pediatric: 0.1 mg/Kg IV, may repeat up to 10 mg
Tricyclic Antidepressants	Sodium bicarbonate	1 mEq/Kg IV repeat PRN

Spinal Nerve Assessment

Dermatomes (sensory)
(Spinal nerve innervations of the skin)

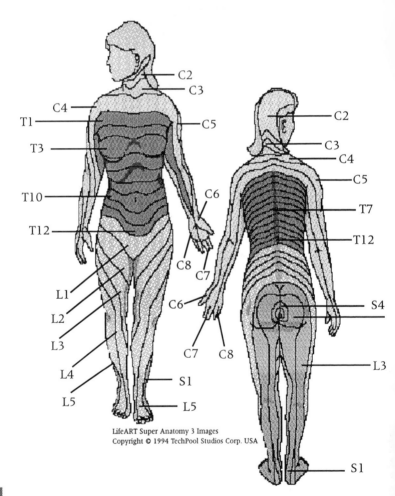

LifeART Super Anatomy 3 Images
Copyright © 1994 TechPool Studios Corp. USA

Spinal Nerve Assessment

Myotomes (Motor)
(Neuromuscular Innervations from the Spinal Nerves)

Motor Nerve Root	Indicates nerve intactness if the patient can:
C2, C3, CN, XI	Shrug their shoulders
C3, C5	Normally breathe, cough
C5	Abduct (raise) their arms above their shoulders
C6	Extend their wrist with palms down
C7	Flex their wrist with palms up
C8 - T1	Spread and close their fingers, make a fist
T2 - T12	(No good test, innervate intercostal muscles)
L1 - L2	Flex their hip (raise their leg)
L3	Straighten out their knee
L4 - L5	Dorsiflex (raise) their big toe
S1	Plantar flex their feet (point their toes)
S2	Curl their toes

Assessment of the Cranial Nerves

No.	CRANIAL NERVE	FUNCTION	INJURY WILL CAUSE:
I	OLFACTORY	Sense of smell	Absence of smell (anosmia)
II	OPTIC	Sight, blink reflex	Visual disturbances
III	OCULOMOTOR	Controls four eye muscles, eyelid, constriction of the pupil	Ptosis, dilated pupil, eye turns down and out
IV	TROCHLEAR	Innervates the eye muscle	Impaired eye movement, cannot move eye down and out
V	TRIGEMINAL	Sensation to face above the eye; the cornea; lips and chin	Loss of sensation of touch (pain) and motor skills
VI	ABDUCENS	Innervates the eye muscle	Inability of the eye to move laterally
VII	FACIAL	Controls muscles of the face, taste on the anterior 2/3 of the tounge	Paralysis of the facial muscles, eye remains open, mouth droops, forehead will fail to wrinkle
VIII	ACOUSTIC	Hearing and equilibrium	Loss of hearing, vertigo, tinnitus
IX	GLOSSOPHARYN-GEAL	Taste on the posterior 1/3 of the tongue, controls swallowing	Loss of taste on posterior 1/3 of tongue, difficulty swallowing
X	VAGUS	Innervates pharynx and larynx, slows smooth & cardiac muscle	Deviation of uvula toward the normal side, hoarseness from paralysis of vocal cords
XI	ACCESSORY	Innervates sternocleido-mastoid and trapezius muscles	Inability to "shrug shoulders"
XII	HYPOGLOSSAL	Movement of tongue	The tongue to protrude toward the affected side

Adult Glasgow Coma Scale

Reassess every 5 minutes. Circle best response and record time.

AREAS OF RESPONSE	POINTS	Initial Time	Time	Time	Time	Time	Time
EYE OPENING							
*Eyes open spontaneously	4	4	4	4	4	4	4
*Eyes open in response to voice	3	3	3	3	3	3	3
*Eyes open in response to pain	2	2	2	2	2	2	2
*No eye opening response	1	1	1	1	1	1	1
BEST VERBAL RESPONSE							
*Oriented, e.g., to person, place, time	5	5	5	5	5	5	5
*Confused, speaks but is disoriented	4	4	4	4	4	4	4
*Inappropriate but comprehensible words	3	3	3	3	3	3	3
*Incomprehensible sounds, no words	2	2	2	2	2	2	2
*None	1	1	1	1	1	1	1
BEST MOTOR RESPONSE							
*Obeys commands to move	6	6	6	6	6	6	6
*Localizes painful stimulus	5	5	5	5	5	5	5
*Withdraws from painful stimulus	4	4	4	4	4	4	4
*Flexion, abnormal decorticate posturing	3	3	3	3	3	3	3
*Extension, abnormal decerebrate posturing	2	2	2	2	2	2	2
*No movement or posturing	1	1	1	1	1	1	1
POSSIBLE POINTS	3-15						
		Points	Points	Points	Points	Points	Points

Adult Glasgow Coma Scale

Score

Major Neurological Injury < 8

Moderate Neurological Injury 9-12

Minor Neurological Injury 13-1

Adult Trauma Scale

During patient evaluation and reassessment, circle best response and record time.

Area of Measurement	Coded Value	Initial Score (Time)	In Route (Time)	In Route (Time)	At Hospital (Time)
Systolic Blood Pressure (mmHg)					
> 89	4	4	4	4	4
76-89	3	3	3	3	3
50-75	2	2	2	2	2
1-49	1	1	1	1	1
0	0	0	0	0	0
Respiratory Rate (Spontaneous Inspiration/ minute)*					
10-29	4	4	4	4	4
> 29	3	3	3	3	3
6-9	2	2	2	2	2
1-5	1	1	1	1	1
0	0	0	0	0	0
Glasgow Coma Scale Score					
13-15	4	4	4	4	4
9-12	3	3	3	3	3
6-8	2	2	2	2	2
4-5	1	1	1	1	1
3	0	0	0	0	0
TOTAL POSSIBLE POINTS	0-12	___ points	___ points	___ points	___ points

*Patient initiated, not artificial ventilation

PUPIL GAUGE

Pupil Gauge (mm)

2	3	4	5	6	7	8	9

Describe pupil reaction to light as the size before light application and then after light application.

Example: Right eye: 7 to 4 after the application of light.

Left eye: 8 to 8 after the application of light.

Burns

Burn "Rule of Nines"

4.5%

4.5%

18%

4.5%   4.5%

9%   9%

4.5%

18%

4.5%   4.5%

1%

9%   9%

9%

4.5%

4.5%

13%

2.5%   2.5%

7%   7%

7%

7%

18%

4.5%   4.5%

8%   8%

7%

18%

4.5%   4.5%

8%   8%

9%

4.5%   4.5%

18%

7%   7%

Estimation of the Percent (%) of Body Surface Area (BSA) Burned from 2nd–3rd Degree Burns Using the "Rule of Nines"

(The patient's palmer surface represents approximately 1%)

Age	Head/Neck Front/Back	Thorax/ Abdomen Front/Back	Arms (each) Front/Back	Legs (each) Front/Back	Genitalia
Adult	4 1/2 / 4 1/2	18 / 18	4 1/2 / 4 1/2	9 / 9	1
10–13	6 1/2 / 6 1/2	16 / 16	4 1/2 / 4 1/2	9 / 9	1
5–9	7 1/2 / 7 1/2	16 / 16	4 1/2 / 4 1/2	8 1/2 /8 1/2	1
1–4	8 1/2 / 8 1/2	17 / 17	4 1/2 / 4 1/2	7 1/2 / 7 1/2	1
Infant (0–1)	9 / 9	18 / 18	4 1/2 / 4 1/2	7 / 7	1

AMERICAN BURN ASSOCIATION BURN SEVERITY CLASSIFICATION

BURN CLASSIFICATION	CHARACTERISTICS
Minor burn injury	1° burns
	2° burn <15% BSA in adults 2° burn < 5% in children/elderly
	3° burn < 2% BSA
Moderate burn injury	2° 15%-25% BSA in adults
	2° burn 10%-20% BSA in children/elderly
	3° burn < 10% BSA
Major burn injury	2° burn > 25% BSA in adults
	2° burn > 20% BSA in children/elderly
	3° burn > 10% BSA
	Burns that involve hands, face, eyes, ears, feet, or perineum.
	Most patients with inhalation injury, electrical injury, concomitant major trauma, or significant pre-existing medical history.

Prehospital Use of the Parkland Burn Formula

The Parkland Burn Formula (derived from the Parkland Hospital; Dallas, Texas)

Four (4) milliliters of IV fluid times the percent of body surface area (BSA) burned (using the "rule of nines") times the patient's weight in kilograms equals the total amount of fluid the patient is to receive in 24 hours.

The patient should receive half (1/2) this amount in the first eight hours using an isotonic solution (0.9% sodium chloride or lactated ringer's) and the remaining half (1/2) of the fluid over the next 16 hours.

> 4 ml x % BSA burned x Kg wt. = fluid to be given over 24 hours. Half of this is given in the first 8 hours and the remaining amount over the last 16 hours.

Prehospital use of the Parkland Burn Formula

Prehospital fluid administration for the burn patient only deals with the first eight (8) hours of the fluid administration. More specifically, the drip rate needs to be known to give the appropriate amount over the eight hours. The prehospital drip rate calculation for the burn formula using a 10 drop per milliliter IV administration set would be:

$$\frac{2 \text{ mL x \% BSA burned x Kg wt. x 10 gtts/mL}}{480 \text{ min (8 hrs)}} = \text{IV drip rate for the first eight hours of the fluid infusion}$$

Example: A 176 pound male with 20% BSA of skin burns should have an IV started of normal saline or lactated Ringer's and the IV drip rate set at 67 gtts/min.

$$\frac{2 \text{ mL x } 20\% \text{ BSA burned x } 80 \text{ Kg x } 10 \text{ gtts/mL}}{480 \text{ min}} = 67 \text{ gtts/min}$$

This formula can be simplified to the following depending on which type of IV administration set is being used (10 gtts/ml set, 15 gtts/ml set, or 20 gtts/ml set).

Using a 10 gtts/mL IV administration set:

$$\frac{\% \text{ BSA burned x Kg wt.}}{24} = \text{gtts/min or ml/hr} \quad (\text{for the first 8 hours})$$

Using a 15 gtts/mL IV administration set:

$$\frac{\% \text{ BSA burned x Kg wt.}}{16} = \text{gtts/min or ml/hr} \quad (\text{for the first 8 hours})$$

Using a 20 gtts/mL IV administration set:

$$\frac{\% \text{ BSA burned x Kg wt.}}{12} = \text{gtts/min or ml/hr} \quad (\text{for the first 8 hours})$$

Oxygen and Ventilation

Oxygen Cylinder Capacities

Minutes of oxygen available in the tank when full at 2200 PSI

Flow Rate	Cylinder Size				
(L/M)	D	E	G	H&K	M
1	320	560	4820	6280	3120
2	160	280	2410	3140	1560
3	106	186	1606	2093	1040
4	80	140	1205	1570	780
5	64	112	964	1256	624
6	53	93	803	1046	520
7	45	80	688	897	445
8	40	70	602	785	390
9	35	62	535	697	346
10	32	56	482	628	312
11	29	50	438	570	283
12	26	46	401	523	260
13	24	43	370	483	240
14	22	40	344	448	222
15	21	37	321	418	208
20	16	28	241	314	156
25	12	22	192	251	124

The amount of oxygen available in an O_2 cylinder can be determined given the tank size, PSI gauge reading, and liter flow delivered to the patient.

$$\frac{\text{(Gauge pressure in PSI - 200 PSI safe residual*) X cylinder factor}}{\text{liter flow per minute}}$$

$$= O_2 \text{ remaining in the cylinder in minutes}$$

Cylinder factors:

D - 0.16   H - 3.14

E - 0.28   K - 3.14

G - 2.41   M -1.56

* Safe residual pressure 200 PSI is the lowest amount of cylinder pressure in PSI that should be left in any O_2 tank. Never run a tank to 0 PSI.

Example: Using a D cylinder containing 2200 PSI gauge reading and delivering 15 liters a minute liter flow to a patient, how long will the oxygen last?

$$\frac{\text{(2200 PSI - 200 PSI safe residual) X 0.16 cylinder factor}}{15 \text{ L/m}}$$

$$= 21 \text{ minutes of } O_2$$

Supplemental Oxygen Delivery Devices

Device	Flow Rate	Oxygen Delivery %
BVM	None	21%
BVM with O_2	12-15 L/M	60%
BVM with O_2 and reservoir	12-15 L/M	90-95%
Demand valve	40-60 L/M	100%
Nasal cannula	1-6 L/M	24-44%
Non rebreather mask	6-15 L/M	60-100%
Pocket mask, O_2	10-15 L/M	21-80%
Simple face mask	8-10 L/M	40-60%
Venturi mask	4 L/M	24%
	4 L/M	28%
	8 L/M	35%
	8 L/M	40%
Automatic transport ventilator (ATV)	15-30 L/M	100%

Suctioning

Type	Suction Setting (-mmHg)
Oral/pharyngeal	-120 to -300 mmHg
Tracheobronchial (ETT) and pediatric suctioning	-80 to -120 mmHg

Pulse Oximetry (Sa0$_2$)

Normal perfusion	97-99%
Inadequate perfusion	91-96% (The patient needs supplemental oxygen)
Poor perfusion	Less than 91%
	(The patient needs aggressive oxygen therapy)

Problems and Corrections of Pulse Oximetry

Factors that affect the reliability of pulse oximetry and ways to correct the problem.

Remember, Sa0$_2$ readings between 70-99% are the most reliable.

Cause of the Error	Problem	Correction
Motion		
Shivering, seizures, vehicle movement	Sensor unable to determine arterial pulsation	Minimize patient movement; move sensor to ear
External Light		
Overhead lights	External light source confuses sensor	Cover sensor with towel
Poor Perfusion States		
Hypovolemia, hypotension, hypothermia, vasoconstriction	Not enough arterial blood flow for sensor to read	Treat the underlying problem; move sensor to ear

Cause of the Error	Problem	Correction
Abnormal Hemoglobin		
Carbon monoxide poisoning	Gives false positive readings; CO binds with hemoglobin better than O_2	Consider the patient's environment, give 100% O_2
Poor Sensor Placement		
Finger clip	Sensor unable to read arterial pulsations	Verify patient's pulse with sensor reading; firmly attach sensor
Venous Pulsations		
Right side heart failure, possibly tension pneumothorax, pericardial tamponade	Back up of venous blood may cause venous pulsation giving false positive readings	Treat the underlying cause
Finger Nail Polish		
Dark colored polishes: black, blue, green	Dark colors can sometimes block sensor light	Remove polish; move sensor to ear

Needle Cricothyrotomy

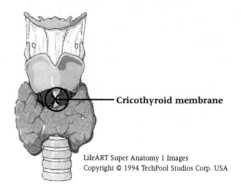

Cricothyroid membrane

LifeART Super Anatomy 1 Images
Copyright © 1994 TechPool Studios Corp. USA

1. Locate the cricoid membrane by sliding a finger down off of the larynx (Adam's apple) to the base where there is a V- or U-like depression.

2. Prep the area with an alcohol prep or iodine swab.

3. Attach a 14 or 16 gauge IV needle to a 12 or 20 ml syringe and aspirate air halfway into the barrel of the syringe.

4. Stabilize the larynx with one hand and insert the IV needle into the cricothyroid membrane at a 90 degree angle to the skin.

5. When a "pop" is felt, advance the needle and catheter slightly while aspirating on the syringe. If air freely flows into the syringe the placement is in the trachea. If no air is aspirated or there is resistance, advance a little deeper until free air is withdrawn.

6. Push the air from the syringe into the trachea. There should be no resistance.

7. Angle the needle down toward the patient's feet and advance the IV catheter up to the hub.

8. Attach a 3 mm pediatric ET tube adapter into the catheter hub.

9. Attach a BVM or demand valve to the ET adapter and begin to ventilate the patient at a ratio of 1 second of ventilation and 4 seconds of exhalation.

10. Attempt to auscultate lung sounds.

Thoracic Needle Decompression (for a Tension Pneumothorax)

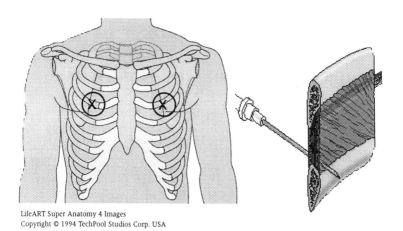

LifeART Super Anatomy 4 Images
Copyright © 1994 TechPool Studios Corp. USA

Figure A

The X marks the needle insertion site.

Figure B

Insert the needle over top of the rib.

1. Determine if the tension pneumothorax is on the right or left side of the patient.

2. Feel for the Angle of Louis (manubrium) on the patient's sternum by sliding a finger down from the suprasternal notch until a slight bump is felt on the sternum. This is the start of the second rib.

3. Slide a finger laterally onto the second rib toward the side of the pneumothorax identifying the mid clavicular line.

4. Slide a finger down to find the third intercostal space in between the second and third rib.

5. This is the location of the needle insertion site. (Figure A)

6. Attach a large bore IV needle (14 or 16 gauge) to the end of a 12 or 20 ml syringe and aspirate air into half of the syringe. (You do not need to use a syringe with the IV needle but it offers better control and ease of insertion. If no syringe is used, remove the cap off the end of the flash chamber on the IV needle to allow air to escape.)

7. With gloves on, prep the insertion site with an alcohol prep, preferably iodine or betadine.

8. Enter the skin with the needle by aiming for the top of the third rib. (Figure B)

9. When the top of the rib is hit, angle the needle slightly upward to slide over the top of the rib.

10. While aspirating on the syringe push the needle into the intercostal muscle and pleural space.

11. A "pop" should be felt as the pleural space is entered, and air should freely aspirate into the syringe. If air is not freely aspirated, the needle and catheter may need to be advanced further. (If there is an increased suction pulling

in on the syringe plunger, the pleural space was not pressurized to begin with.)

12. If the plunger aspirates freely, remove the plunger completely from the barrel of the syringe. There should be a hiss of air as the pressure escapes.

13. Advance the needle and catheter slightly into the chest wall and then advance the catheter to the hub while removing the needle and syringe.

14. An attempt to attach a finger cot to the hub of the catheter may be made, but this is more easily done in theory than in practice. Although the thorax is "open," by leaving the hub open, you still allow for pressurized air to be released and a simple pneumothorax is not life threatening.

15. Minimize the patient's movement, especially the arm on the side of the chest in which the catheter is placed. Too much chest wall/muscle movement can pinch off the catheter.

16. Continually reassess for the redevelopment of a tension pneumothorax on that side.

Hazardous Materials and Radiation Emergencies

Hazardous Material Placards
International Placards and Color Codes

Color Code	Hazardous Classification
Green	Nonflammable gas
Orange	Explosive
Red	Flammable
White	Poison
White over black	Corrosive
White and red stripes	Flammable solid
Yellow	Oxidizer/Peroxide
Yellow over white	Radioactive

International Hazardous Material Placard Classification Codes

Class or division numbers should be displayed in the bottom of placards or on the shipping papers. In certain cases, a class or division number will replace the written name of the hazardous material in the shipping papers. The class and division numbers mean the following:

Class 1 Explosives

Division 1.1	Explosives with a mass explosion hazard
Division 1.2	Explosives with a projection hazard
Division 1.3	Explosives with predominantly a fire hazard
Division 1.4	Explosives with no significant blast hazard
Division 1.5	Very insensitive explosives
Division 1.6	Extremely insensitive explosive articles

Class 2 Gases

Division 2.1	Flammable gases
Division 2.2	Nonflammable gases
Division 2.3	Poison gases
Division 2.4	Corrosive gases (Canadian)

Class 3 Flammable Liquids

Division 3.1	Flash point below - 18° C (0° F)
Division 3.2	Flash point - 18° C and above but less than 23° C (73° F)
Division 3.3	Flash point of 23° C and up to 61° C (141°F)

Class 4 Flammable solids, spontaneously combustible materials, materials that are dangerous when wet

Division 4.1	Flammable solids
Division 4.2	Spontaneously combustible materials
Division 4.3	Materials that are dangerous when wet

Class 5 Oxidizers and Organic Peroxides

Division 5.1	Oxidizers
Division 5.2	Organic peroxides

Class 6 Poisonous and Etiological Materials

Division 6.1	Poisonous materials
Division 6.2	Etiological materials

Class 7 Radioactive Materials

Class 8 Corrosives

Class 9 Miscellaneous Hazardous Materials

Placards with four (4) digit numbers in the middle of the plac-
ard define specific substances and represent US DOT reference
numbers as to the content.

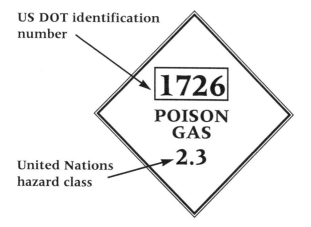

US DOT identification number

United Nations hazard class

Radiation Emergencies
Radiation Color Code Classifications Chart

Placard	Radiation Exposure	
Color Code	**Distance: Next to source**	**Distance: 3 ft. away**
White I	Less than 0.5 mR per hour (Low to almost no radiation)	Minimal
Yellow II	0.5-50 mR per hour (Low to medium radiation)	Less than 1 mR per hour
Yellow III	50-200 mR per hour (Medium to high radiation)	1-10 mR per hour

(mR = milli Roentgen)

Radiation Absorbed Dose (RAD)

Radiation dose Equivalent in Man (REM)

Roentgen/hour = Rad/hour = Rem/hour

Emergency Phone Numbers for Radiation Accidents

Agency for Toxic Substances and Disease Registry (ATSDR)	24 hour consultation for the treatment of chemically contaminated patients	(404) 639-6360
Chemtrec	24 hour information emergency response to transported chemicals	(800) 424-9300
National Response Center (NRC)	24 hour information for identifying hazardous materials	(800) 424-8802

| Nuclear Regulatory Commission (NRC) | 24 hour information on emergency response to radioactive materials | (301) 951-0550 |
| Radiation Emergency Assistance Center/ Training Site (REAC/TS) | 24 hour information on emergency response and treatment of radioactive patients | (423) 576-3131 (423) 481-1000 (after hours) |

SECTION TEN

Medication Math Calculations and Medication Abbreviations and Equivalents

Math Calculations

Rule of 10% for converting the patient's weight in pounds to kilograms:

Take half (1/2) of the patient's weight in pounds and multiply that number by 10%. Then subtract the 10% number from the halved patient weight in pounds to equal the patient's weight in kilograms.

Patient weight in lbs = **(a) x 10% = (b).**
$\quad$ **2**
Then (a) - (b) = (c)
(c) = patient's weight in kilograms

Example: $\underline{160 \text{ lbs}}$ = 80 x 10% = 8.
$\qquad$ 2
Then 80 - 8 = 72 Kg. 160 lbs = 72 kgs.

Fluid Administration Math:

The amount of fluid to be infused in milliliters multiplied by the drip factor of the IV administration set in drops per milliliter (gtts/ml) divided by the time in minutes the fluid is to be administered equals the drops per minute the IV should be set at.

Amount of fluid (ml) x gtts/ml
IV administration set = **gtts/minute**
$\quad$ **Time (in minutes)**

Example:
$\underline{500 \text{ ml x 10 gtts/ml set up}}$ = $\underline{500 \text{ ml x 10 gtts/cc}}$ = 41.6 or 42 gtts/min.
$\quad$ 2 hrs or (2x60 min) = Time 120 minutes
$\quad$ in mins.

Medication administration math for IV push medications, intramuscular, subcutaneous, intradermal, and sublingual injections:

You must know the physician or protocol order of the drug, how the drug is supplied, and the patient's weight in pounds.

Step 1. Make all of the conversions of the drug order first:

> **1a.** Convert the patient's weight in pounds (lbs) to kilograms (Kgs)(if necessary) using the 10% rule for converting lbs to Kgs.

> $$\frac{160 \text{ lbs}}{2} = 80 \times 10\% = 8. \text{ Then } 80 - 8 = 72 \text{ kgs.}$$

> **1b.** Convert the drug unit weight into the unit weight of the physician or protocol order. (Gms to mgs, mgs to mcgs, or Gms to mcgs).

> The doctor orders 250 mgs IV push. The drug supply is 1 gm in 10 mls.

> 1 Gm = 1000 mgs, so 1 Gm in 10 mls equals 1000 mgs in 10 mls.

Step 2. Divide the supply weight of the drug from step 1b by the volume of the supply in milliliters to determine the concentration of the drug per one milliliter.

> $\frac{Gm}{mL}$ or $\frac{mg}{mL}$ or $\frac{mcg}{mL}$ = the concentration of the drug per one milliliter.

> $$\frac{1000 \text{ mgs}}{10 \text{ mls}} = 100 \text{ mgs in 1 ml or 100 mgs/ml.}$$

Step 3. Multiply the drug order by the patient's weight in kilograms (if part of the order) and divide this by the concentration of the drug supply from Step 2 which then equals the amount of milliliters to be administered.

$$\frac{250 \text{ mgs}}{100 \text{ mgs/ml}} = 2.5 \text{ mls to be administered}$$

Example:
Physician/protocol order: Give 5 mg/Kg of drug Z IV push. Drug Z is supplied: 1 gram in 10 ml ampules. Patient weighs 160 lbs.

Step 1a. 160 lbs = 72 Kg

Step 1b. 1 gram/10 ml = 1000 mg/10 ml

Step 2. Concentration : $\frac{1000 \text{ mg}}{10 \text{ ml}}$ = 100 mg/ml

Step 3. $\frac{\text{Dr. order x Kg}}{\text{Concentration}}$

or

$$\frac{5 \text{ mg x 72 Kg}}{100 \text{ mg/ml}} = \frac{360 \text{ mg}}{100 \text{ mg/ml}} = 3.6 \text{ ml to be administered}$$

Example:
Physician/protocol order: Give 8 mg IM of drug Z. Drug Z is supplied: 20 mg in 5 ml ampules. Patient weighs 160 lbs.

Step 1a. None (order does not require patient weight)

Step 1b. None (supply weight of drug is the same as the order weight)

Step 2. Concentration - $\underline{20\ mg} = 4\ mg/ml$
$5\ ml$

Step 3. $\underline{8\ mg} = 2\ mls$ to be administered
$4\ mg/ml$

Medication infusion math for IV infusions and drips

You must know the physician or protocol order of the amount of drug to be administered, the mixture of the solution, how the drug is supplied, and the patient weight in pounds.

Step 1. Make all of the conversions of the drug order first:

1a. Convert the patient's weight in pounds (lbs) to kilograms (Kgs)(if necessary) using the 10% rule for converting lbs to Kgs.

$\underline{160\ lbs} = 80 \times 10\% = 8$. Then $80 - 8 = 72$ kgs.
2

1b. Convert the drug unit weight into the drug unit weight of the physician or protocol order (Gms to mgs, mgs to mcgs, or Gms to mcgs).

The physician orders a 2 mg per minute IV drip. The drug supply is 1 Gm in 10 mls. 1 Gm equals 1000 mgs, so 1 Gm in 10 mls equals 1000 mgs in 10 mls.

Step 2. Determine the concentration of the IV mixture per ml when adding the medication to the IV fluid bag by dividing the weight of the drug added to fluid (using the number from Step 1b) by the amount of IV fluid being used.

$$\frac{\text{Drug supply weight}}{\text{Amount of IV fluid}} = \text{Drug weight per one milliliter}$$

$$\frac{1000 \text{ mgs in 10 ml}}{250 \text{ mls normal saline}} = 4 \text{ mgs/ml}$$

Note: The 10 mls in the drug supply is dropped in the calculation. Technically, when adding the medication to the IV bag, the 10 mls in the drug supply would make the total amount of fluid in the IV bag 260 mls.

Step 3. Multiply the physician's order by the patient's weight in kilograms (if part of the order) and by the IV administration set being used (either 60 gtts/mL or 10 gtts/mL) and divide this by the concentration in the IV fluid bag from Step 2.

$$\frac{\text{Drs. order x IV administration set}}{\text{Concentration in the IV bag}} = \text{Drops per minute or gtts/min.}$$

$$\frac{2 \text{ mgs/min x 60 gtts/ml}}{4 \text{ mgs/ml}} = 30 \text{ gtts/minute drip rate}$$

Example:
Physician/protocol order: 2 mcg/Kg/min of drug Z using a 60 gtts/mL IV administration set.

Mix: 400 mgs of drug Z into 500 ml normal saline (NS)
The patient weighs 160 lbs.
Drug Z is supplied: 400 mg in 10 ml prefilled syringes

Step 1a. 160 lbs = 72 Kg

Step 1b. Physician/protocol order is in micrograms and the drug is supplied in milligrams. Convert milligrams to micrograms:

400 mgs/10 mls = 400,000 mcgs/10 mls (1 mg = 1000 mcg)

Step 2. Determine the concentration in the IV fluid bag after adding the 400,000 mcg/10 ml into the 500 ml IV fluid.

$$\frac{400,000 \text{ mcg/10 ml}}{500 \text{ mls NS}} = 800 \text{ mcgs/ml concentration}$$

(Note - The 10 ml supply volume is not added into the total amount of fluid in the IV bag)

Step 3. Physician/protocol order multiplied by the patient weight in Kgs times 60 gtts/mL IV administration set divided by the concentration in the IV bag from Step 2.

$$\frac{2 \text{ mcg x 72 Kgs x 60 gtts/ml}}{800 \text{ mcg/ml}} = 10.8 \text{ or 11 gtts/minute drip rate}$$

Common Medication Abbreviations and Equivalents

Abbreviations		Equivalents
Kg	Kilogram	1 Kilogram = 1,000 G
G (gm)	Gram	1 Gram = 1,000 mg
mg	Milligram	1 Milligram = 0.001 G
mcg	Microgram	1 Milligram = 1,000 mcg
lb	Pound	1 Microgram = 0.001 mg
oz	Ounce (weight)	1 Grain = 60 mg
gr	Grain	1 Milligram = 1/60 grain
mEq	Milliequivalent	1 Liter = 1,000 ml
L	Liter	1 Milliliter = 0.001 liters
ml (mL)	Milliliter	1 Fluid ounce = 30 ml
cc	Cubic centimeter	1 Tablespoon = 15 ml
oz (fl. oz.)	Ounce (fluid)	1 Teaspoon = 5 ml
tbsp	Tablespoon	1 Cubic centimeter = 1 ml
tsp	Teaspoon	1 Liter = 1.05 quarts
gtt(s)	Drop(s)	1 Kilogram = 2.2 pounds
prn	As needed	
po	By mouth	
pr (PR)	By rectum	
q	Every	
IM	Intramuscular	
IO	Intraosseous	
IV	Intravenous	

Abbreviations

KVO	Keep vein open
min	Minute
mg/ml	Milligram(s) per milliliter
gtt/ml	Number of drops to provide one milliliter
gtts/min	Rate of IV fluid administration, drops per minute
SQ, Sub-Q	Subcutaneous
SL	Sublingual
TKO	To keep open

Temperature Conversion

To convert Fahrenheit to Celsius (Centigrade):

5/9 (Fahrenheit minus 32) = Celsius

To convert Celsius to Fahrenheit:

9/5 (Celsius plus 32) = Fahrenheit

Accessing Vascular Access Devices (VAD's)

Accessing Vascular Access Devices (VAD's)

Vascular access devices (VAD's) are long-term implantable catheters which are placed into a patient's central venous circulation for repeated venous access. Numerous patients are being discharged from the hospital with these devices in place so that home health care can be provided instead of long hospital stays. These devices can be accessed by prehospital personnel in emergency situations where normal peripheral IV cannulation cannot be obtained. There are three types of VAD's that may be encountered and used as an IV site.

TYPES

Implantable (Mediports)

Peripheral inserted central catheters (PICC's)

Central venous catheters (CVC's)

Implantable VAD's (Mediports)

Implantable VAD's (Mediports) are small reservoirs implanted just below the skin, in the anticubital area of the arm, the lower chest wall, or the upper chest wall, below the clavicles. The reservoir has a self-sealing port just below the skin surface for needle access. These ports are designed to be punctured with a "Huber" needle but a regular needle (21 gauge or smaller) can be used in an emergency.

Emergency Access of an Implantable VAD (Mediport)

1. Palpate the device with the fingers. It will feel like a small hard disk beneath the skin.

2. Clean the site with an alcohol prep, preferably with an iodine or betadine prep using spiral motions - inside to outside.

3. Attach a 21 gauge or smaller needle to a 12 ml syringe that has been filled halfway (6 ml) with normal saline.

4. With sterile gloves on, stretch the skin over top of the reservoir.

5. Inject the needle directly into the center of the reservoir through the skin at a 90 degree angle. (There will be quite a bit of resistance going through the scar tissue and the port.)

6. Insert the needle until it hits the bottom of the reservoir.

7. Aspirate for free flowing blood into the syringe. (If no blood is aspirated, reposition the patient by rolling them side to side, raising their arm, or if the VAD is in the patient's anticubital area, bending or straightening the arm slightly.)

8. If there is a blood return, inject the saline/blood back into the reservoir to verify a free flowing catheter.

9. Disconnect the syringe from the needle and attach the IV tubing as quickly as possible to prevent air from entering the VAD.

10. The needle will probably stand straight up on its own. Secure the IV tubing to the patient. Gauze rolls can be used to support the needle.

Peripheral Inserted Central Catheters (PICC's)

Peripheral inserted central catheters (PICC's) are small diameter catheters that are inserted into easily accessible veins such as in the arm or anticubital area. Because of their small size, they are used frequently in children. They are not typically used for long-term placement but patients may be sent home with them in place for short-term home health care use. They may be single or double lumen (port) catheters, but most often single lumen. The ports usually have a cap covering the catheter hub or if they are in use, some type of IV tubing will be attached.

Central Venous Catheters (CVC's)
(Broviac, Groshong, Hickman)

Central venous catheters (CVC's) are long-term indwelling catheters that are placed into a central vein such as the subclavian with the tip inserted directly into the right atrium of the heart. CVC's typically are referred to by the manufacturer's name of the device as listed above. These catheters, like the PICC lines, may have multiple lumens. The CVC ports are usually found near the patient's clavicle or on their chest wall. The lumen ports have a cap covering the catheter hub, or if they are in use, some type of IV tubing attached.

Emergency Access of PICC or CVC Lines

1. Locate the catheter lumen. If the patient is receiving medication from an IV pump, stop the infusion.

2. If there are multiple lumens, the venous catheter lumen should be blue in color.

3. Clamp the catheter closed by using the V-clamp attached to the tubing or fold the tubing over to occlude it. If hemostats are being used, use those that are smooth and without teeth to avoid damaging the catheter.

4. Prepare a 12 ml syringe containing 6 ml of normal saline.

5. Prepare an IV bag and tubing insuring that the line is completely flushed.

6. With sterile gloves on, carefully clean the cap and lumen with an alcohol prep, preferably with iodine or betadine.

7. Remove the cap from the lumen and attach the syringe. If a needleless IV system is being used, the syringe can be inserted with a connector directly into the cap. Unclamp the catheter.

8. Aspirate blood into the syringe. If a free flow of blood is not obtained move the patient by rolling them from side to side, have them raise their arms or cough to attempt to move the catheter tip in the atrium. Do not aspirate so hard as to collapse or damage the catheter.

9. With a free flow of blood into the syringe, push the blood/saline back into the line to ensure patency.

10. Clamp the line again (to prevent an air embolism) and attach the IV tubing to the lumen.

11. Unclamp the catheter and adjust the flow of the IV fluid.

12. Secure the IV tubing to the patient.

Intravenous Fluid Information

0.9% Sodium Chloride
(0.9% NaCl) "Normal Saline"

Classification:	Isotonic crystalloid solution
Actions:	Volume expansion
Indications:	Hypovolemia, volume replacement, diabetic ketoacidosis, crush injuries, dehydration, eye irrigation, freshwater drowning with aspiration, heat exhaustion, heat stroke, head injuries
Contraindications:	(Relative): Congestive heart failure, pulmonary edema, renal failure
Precautions:	Volume overload
Side Effects:	Volume overload, hypothermia with large infusions; depletion of electrolytes following large infusions, hyperchloremia, metabolic acidosis
Route of Administration:	IV infusion, intraosseous infusion
Dosage (Adult):	Burns: use the Parkland Burn Formula Trauma: 1-2 liters initially and then titrate to effect
Dosage (Pediatric):	20 mL/Kg bolus titrate to effect

0.45% Sodium Chloride
(0.45% NaCl) "Half Normal Saline"

Classification:	Hypotonic crystalloid solution
Actions:	Sodium and chloride electrolyte replacement
Indications:	Slow replacement of sodium and chloride electrolytes in hemodynamically stable patients with compromised renal or cardiovascular status
Contraindications:	Do not use when volume expansion is indicated in the unstable patient (consider 0.9% NaCl)
Precautions:	Rare, if used for appropriate indications
Side Effects:	Depletion of electrolytes following large infusions of 0.45% NS
Route of Administration:	IV infusion, intraosseous infusion
Dosage (Adult):	Titrated to effect
Dosage (Pediatric):	Titrated to effect

Lactated Ringer's Solution

Classification:	Isotonic crystalloid solution
Actions:	Cardiovascular volume expander
Indications:	Burns, hypovolemia, dehydration, crush injuries
Contraindications:	Congestive heart failure, pulmonary edema, closed head injuries
Precautions:	Watch for volume overload
Side Effects:	Volume overload and hypothermia with large infusions
Route of Administration:	IV infusion, intraosseous infusion
Dosage (Adult):	Burns: use the Parkland Burn Formula Trauma: 1-2 liters initially and then titrate to effect
Dosage (Pediatric):	20 ml/Kg bolus titrated to effect

5% Dextrose in Water (D5W)

Classification:	A hypotonic solution of sugar and water
Actions:	Glucose and water additive solution
Indications:	Administration solution for IV medications and infusions
Contraindications:	Should not to be used as volume expander Avoid starting an IV using D5W in seizure patients because Dilantin (phenytoin) cannot be given through D5W
Precautions:	None if used as indicated
Side Effects:	Hyperglycemia; may exacerbate cerebral edema in patients suffering from head injury or stroke
Route of Administration:	IV infusion, intraosseous infusion
Dosage (Adult):	Titrated to effect
Dosage (Pediatric):	Avoid using in the pediatric patient; glucose-containing solutions can cause dehydration by renal excretion of high serum glucose levels

Emergency Medication Information

Activated Charcoal

Trade Name:	Acta-char, Intsa-char, Liqui-char
Generic Name:	Activated charcoal
Classification:	Absorbent
Actions:	Prevents gastrointestinal absorption of a variety of drugs and chemicals
Indications:	Treatment for oral poisonings and overdoses of oral medications
Contraindications:	Do not use with petroleum or corrosive ingestions. Patient must be awake and alert for oral administration.
Side Effects:	Constipation, diarrhea, and vomiting
Route of Administration:	Oral (the patient will need to drink the solution), or by a nasogastric tube
Dosage Range (Adult):	50-100 grams, mixed with a glass of water or juice to form a slurry. Do not mix with milk.
Dosage Range (Pediatric):	1 gram/Kg mixed with a glass of water to form a slurry
Supplied:	Powder form for mixing with water

Special Considerations: Should be administered following emesis for the greatest effect unless emesis is contraindicated or not desired. Activated charcoal does not absorb cyanide or organic solvents and has poor absorption of ethanol, methanol, and iron.

Adenosine
(ah-den'oh-seen)

Trade Name: Adenocard

Generic Name: Adenosine

Classification: Antiarrhythmic

Actions: Transiently blocks conduction through the AV node

Indications: Converts supraventricular tachycardia (SVT) including WPW syndrome. Does not convert atrial fibrillation, atrial flutter, or ventricular arrhythmias.

Contraindications: Sick sinus syndrome, heart blocks, and bradycardias. Patients taking dipyridamole (Persantine) which blocks the breakdown of adenosine. Use caution with patients who have had a heart transplant.

Side Effects: Chest pain, SOB, and facial flushing. Will cause a transient heart block. Also may cause transient arrhythmias during conversion from PSVT to sinus rhythm - which may include ventricular tachycardia or asystole. These side effects are usually limited due to the short half life of this drug (less than 10 seconds).

Route of Administration: Rapid IV push - followed by a 20 ml saline flush

Dosage Range (Adult): 6 mg rapid IV push given over 1-2 seconds. May repeat within 2 minutes at 12 mg if not converted. May repeat the 12 mg dose one time.

Dosage Range (Pediatric): 0.1 mg/Kg (max 6 mg) rapid IV and IO. May repeat within 2 minutes at 0.2 mg/Kg (max 12 mg).

Supplied: 6 mg/2 ml and 12 mg/2 ml vials, prefilled syringes

Special Considerations: Have the patient on a monitor and insure that the IV line is patent. Administer the drug through the IV port closest to the patient followed by a rapid saline flush. Begin recording the EKG before administering the bolus of adenosine.

Albuterol
(al-byoo'ter-ole)

Trade Name:	Proventil, Ventolin
Generic Name:	Albuterol
Classification:	Bronchodilator, sympathomimetic
Actions:	Selective beta 2 adrenergic bronchodilator
Indications:	Bronchial asthma, reversible bronchospasms associated with chronic bronchitis or emphysema, and wheezing
Contraindications:	Patients with a history of hypersensitivity to the drug, tachyarrhythmias
Side Effects:	Tremors, dizziness, nervousness, headaches, anxiety, palpitations, nausea
Route of Administration:	Aerosolized inhalation using 6-10 LPM O_2 flow
Dosage Range (Adult):	3 ml (2.5 mg) mixed in 2 ml NS by nebulization until medication is gone. May repeat up to 3 total doses.
Dosage Range (Pediatric):	<u>2 years of age and older:</u> same as an adult dose <u>Less than 2 years of age:</u> give 1/2 the adult dose, 1.5 ml (1.25 mg)

Supplied:	2.5 mg in 3 ml plastic ampules or containers
Special Considerations:	May not be effective if the patient is taking a beta blocker. Has occasionally been reported to cause bronchospasms. Monitor the patient's pulse and blood pressure during administration.

Ammonia Inhalant

Trade Name:	Aromatic Ammonia
Generic Name:	Ammonia inhalant
Classification:	Respiratory irritant, noxious CNS stimulant
Actions:	Local, respiratory mucosa irritant with subsequent CNS noxious stimulation
Indications:	To stimulate a patient who is unresponsive from an unknown cause
Contraindications:	Hypertension, stroke; head injury, patients with respiratory difficulty or distress
Side Effects:	Burning of the respiratory mucosa, respiratory distress, increased blood pressure
Route of Administration:	Inhalation
Dosage Range (Adult):	1 ampule placed 2 to 3 inches from nostrils

Dosage Range (Pediatric): Should not be used

Supplied: Ampules/pearls of ammonia

Special Considerations: Ammonia is a potent irritant to the eyes, nose, and mouth and may cause bronchospasms.

Amyl Nitrate
(am'il ni'trait)

Trade Name: Vaporole

Generic Name: Amyl nitrate

Classification: Antianginal, nitrate

Actions: Amyl nitrate is a coronary vasodilator and a smooth muscle relaxant. In cyanide poisoning, the nitrate combines with hemoglobin in the blood to form methemoglobin to prevent binding with cyanide.

Indications: Cyanide posioning

Contraindications: None if used for cyanide poisoning

Side Effects: Hypotension and tachycardia. Alcohol ingestion intensifies the side effects.

Route of Administration: Inhalation. Break one ampule in a guaze pad and hold it to the patient's nose and mouth for 30 seconds, intermittently administering oxygen every 30 seconds. Repeat this combination until the amyl nitrate smell is gone or until sodium nitrate IV is available.

Dosage Range (Adult): 0.3 ml ampules repeated as directed above

Supplied: 0.3 ml ampules

Special Considerations: Has tendency for abuse. Has a very offensive odor.

Aspirin
(as'pir-in)
Acetylsalicylic Acid (ASA)

Trade Name: Bufferin, Empirin, Halfprin, Sloprin

Generic Name: Aspirin

Classification: Antipyretic, analgesic, antiplatelet

Actions: Reduces platelet aggregation to minimize myocardial infarct size. Will also increase bleeding times. Onset of action 5-30 minutes with peak effect between 15 minutes and 2 hours.

Indications:	New onset chest pain considered to be cardiac in origin
Contraindications:	Bleeding disorders including active GI bleeds and stomach ulcers. Hypersensitivity to salicylates.
Side Effects:	Nausea, vomiting, GI bleeding, peptic ulcers, rash, urticaria and bronchospasm. Toxic levels (>300 mcg/ml), tinnitus, headache, dizziness, confusion, hyperpyrexia, and metabolic acidosis.
Route of Administration:	PO
Dosage Range (Adult):	160 to 325 mg
Dosage Range (Pediatric):	Do not use
Supplied:	325 mg tablets, 81 mg (baby aspirin) tablets
Special Considerations:	Not to be used for fever reduction in children with varicella (chicken pox) or influenza due to the increased risk of Reye's syndrome.

Atropine Sulfate
(a'troe-peen súl-fate)

Trade Name:	None
Generic Name:	Atropine sulfate
Classification:	Parasympatholytic, anticholinergic

Actions: Atropine blocks the action of
acetylcholine (ACh) at the
neuromuscular junction of the
parasympathetic nervous system which increases the conduction through the SA and
AV nodes of the heart. With
organophosphate poisoning,
atropine competes for post
synaptic receptors at neuromuscular and neuro-glandular
junctions which block the
action of the poison.

Indications: Symptomatic bradycardias
induced by increased vagal
tone including sinus bradycardia, lst, 2nd, and 3rd degree
AV heart blocks, bradycardic
PEA, and asystole.
Organophosphate poisoning.

Contraindications: Hypertension, tachycardia.
Use with caution in 2nd
degree Type II heart blocks
and wide complex 3rd degree
heart blocks where paradoxical bradycardia may occur and
worsen the block.

Side Effects: Paradoxical bradycardias may
occur if less than 0.5 mg is
given or if given too slowly.
Pupil dilation, dry mouth,
blurred vision, tachycardiac
arrhythmias.

Route of Administration: Rapid IV, transtracheal (ETT), rapid IO

Dosage Range (Adult): Bradycardias - IV: 0.5 mg initial dose, may repeat at 1.0 mg every 3-5 minutes up to a total of 2.5 mg or 0.03 mg/Kg. Asystole or bradycardiac PEA - IV: 1 mg IV every 3-5 minutes up to 3 mg or 0.04 mg/Kg.

Endotracheal tube (ETT): 1-2 mg in 10 mL of normal saline.

Organophosphate poisoning - IV: 2-10 mg until the respiratory status improves.

Dosage Range (Pediatric): Bradycardia (after no response to 2-3 rounds of epinephrine): 0.02 mg/Kg IV, IO (minimum IV, IO dose 0.1 mg)

Children less than 5 years old: maximum single dose 0.5 mg, maximum total dose 1.0 mg

Children over 5 years old: maximum single dose 1.0 mg, maximum total dose 2.0 mg

ETT dose: 0.04 to 0.06 mg/Kg (minimum ETT dose 0.15 mg)

Supplied: Prefilled syringes containing 1 mg/10 ml, 0.5 mg/5 ml ampules of 1 mg/1ml

Special Considerations: IV and IO atropine should be followed by 20 ml saline flush. Atropine may be reversed with physostigmine (Antilirium).

Bretylium Tosylate
(bre-til'ee-um to-sol'ate)

Trade Name: Bretylate, Bretylol

Generic Name: Bretylium tosylate

Classification: Antiarrhythmic

Actions: Bretylol raises the fibrillation threshold level in myocardial cells as well as blocks the release of norepinephrine.

Indications: Bretylol is the second line drug of choice after lidocaine for the treatment of ventricular fibrillation (VF) and ventricular tachycardia (VT).

Contraindications: None if used in the above two situations

Side Effects: Nausea, vomiting, and hypotension may occur if used in a conscious patient. Bretylol should be given slowly in a diluted solution for conscious patients in ventricular tachycardia with a pulse.

Route of Administration: IV, IV infusion, IO

Dosage Range (Adult):

<u>Pulseless ventricular tachycardia or ventricular fibrillation</u>: 5 mg/Kg IV repeated at 10 mg/Kg every 5 minutes up to 35 mg/Kg total dose.

<u>Ventricular tachycardia with a pulse</u>: mix 5-10 mg/Kg in 50 ml NS and infuse over 10 minutes using a 10 gtt/ml IV administration set infusing at 50 gtt/min.

<u>IV maintenance infusion for post conversion</u>: 1-2 mg/min.

Dosage Range (Pediatric): Same as the adult

Drip Mixture (Adult, Peds): 500 mg in 250 ml NS or 1000 mg in 500 ml NS giving a 2 mg/ml concentration for the IV maintenance infusion

Supplied: 500 mg/10 ml ampules and vials

Special Considerations: IV doses should be followed by a 20 ml saline flush. Bretylol may worsen digitalis toxicity and may be incompatible with procainamide.

Calcium Chloride

Trade Name: None
Generic Name: Calcium chloride

Classification:	Electrolyte replacement agent
Actions:	Contraction of cardiac, skeletal, and smooth muscle
Indications:	Rapid replacement of calcium in patients with hypocalemia (decreased calcium) or patients with hyperkalemia (increased potassium). Antidote for calcium channel blocker toxicity (verapamil), toxic bites from black widow spiders, and hydrofluoric acid exposure.
Contraindications:	Use with caution in patients taking digitalis or other cardiac glycosides
Side Effects:	Bradycardia, asystole, ventricular fibrillation, and hypotension with rapid injection
Route of Administration:	IV slow push, IO
Dosage Range (Adult):	2-4 mg/Kg of a 10% solution slow IV push. May be repeated at 10 minute intervals.
Dosage Range (Pediatric):	5-7 mg/Kg of a 10% solution slow IV push, IO
Supplied:	10 ml of a 10% solution (1 gram) prefilled syringes
Special Considerations:	Flush the IV line in between using calcium chloride and sodium bicarbonate.

Extravasation of the IV will
cause tissue necrosis.

Dexamethasone
(dex-a-meth'a-sone)

Trade Name:	Decadron, Hexadrol
Generic Name:	Dexamethasone
Classification:	Anti-inflammatory agent, steroid
Actions:	Dexamethasone is an anti-inflammatory glucocorticoid which strengthens and stablizes white blood cell wall membranes during allergic reactions. This prevents cells from leaking vasodilatory chemicals such as histamine and kinins which can cause edema and fluid shifts in the vasculature.
Indications:	Severe allergic reations, anaphylactic shock, acute asthma attacks
Contraindications:	Hypersensitivity
Side Effects:	Hypotension if given too rapidly; seizures, headache
Route of Administration:	IV slow push
Dosage Range (Adult):	0.1 mg/Kg to 0.25 mg/Kg

Dosage Range (Pediatric):	Same as the adult
Supplied:	4 mg/1 ml vials
Special Considerations:	May be used for spinal cord injuries in some protocols.

50% Dextrose
(dex'tros)

Trade Name:	D50, Insta-Glucose (oral preparation)
Generic Name:	50% Dextrose
Classification:	Carbohydrate
Actions:	Raises circulating serum glucose levels. Acts transiently as an osmotic diuretic.
Indications:	Symptomatic hypoglycemia. Comas of unknown origin.
Contraindications:	None, if documented hypoglycemia exists
Side Effects:	Tissue necrosis if it infiltrates the skin. May precipitate severe neurological symptoms (Wernicke's syndrome) in alcoholics.
Route of Administration:	IV
Dosage Range (Adult):	50 ml of 50% dextrose (25 Gm). May be repeated if there is no response or a minimal response is noted in marked hypoglycemia.

Dosage Range (Pediatric):

<u>Neonate to 1 year:</u> 2-4 ml/Kg of a 10% dextrose solution

To make a 10% dextrose solution, squirt out 40 ml of D50 and replace it with 40 ml of normal saline or sterile water.

<u>1 year to 10 years:</u> 2-4 ml/Kg of a 25% dextrose solution

To make a 25% dextrose solution, squirt out 25 ml of D50 and replace it with 25 ml of normal saline or sterile water.

Supplied:

Prefilled syringes containing 50 ml of 50% Dextrose (25 Gm)

Special Considerations:

Administer through a free flowing IV line, preferably started in a large vein. Tissue necrosis can be extremely severe. Notify the physician immediately on arrival to the hospital if infiltration is suspected. If available, a glucometer blood glucose level should be done prior to administration of dextrose. Use oral glucose only in conscious alert patients with a gag reflex.

Diazepam
(dye-az'e-pam)

Trade Name:	Valium
Generic Name:	Diazepam
Classification:	Anticonvulsant, benzodiazepine
Actions:	Diazepam crosses the blood-brain barrier into the cerebral motor cortex to suppress seizure activity and cause CNS slowing. It will stop active seizures, but it does not prevent them. Diazepam does not have any analgesic properties.
Indications:	Uncontrolled major motor seizures, status epilepticus, acute anxiety, sedation prior to cardioversion, or sedation while using transcutaneous pacing.
Contraindications:	Hypotension, respiratory depression, history of hypersensitivity, alcohol intoxication
Side Effects:	Respiratory depression and arrest, hypotension
Route of Administration:	IV slow push. Rectally in children.
Dosage Range (Adult):	<u>Seizures</u>: 2-10 mg IV until seizure stops

	Anxiety and sedation: 2-5 mg IV
Dosage Range (Pediatric):	IV: 0.2-0.3 mg/Kg up to 5 mg
	Rectal: 0.5 mg/Kg up to 10 mg
Supplied:	10 mg/2 ml (5 mg/ml) ampules and prefilled syringes
Special Considerations:	When using Valium, have airway equipment ready. Monitor the patient's blood pressure during and after administration. Avoid administering through small veins. Inject into the closest IV port possible (diazepam can react with the IV tubing). Flumazenil (Romazican) can reverse sedative effects of diazepam as well as some of the respiratory depression.

Diphenhydramine HCl
(dye-fen-hye'dra-meen)

Trade Name:	Benadryl, Benylin
Generic Name:	Diphenhydramine HCl
Classification:	Antihistamine
Actions:	Diphenhydramine blocks Histamine from reacting with H1 and H2 receptors in the bloodstream during allergic reactions.

Indications:	Anaphylaxis, allergic reactions
Contraindications:	Acute asthmatic attack (because it dries up mucus plugs), hypotension, and pregnancy
Side Effects:	Drowsiness, confusion, hypotension, dry mouth, wheezing, and palpitations. In large doses, tachycardia and hypertension may occur.
Route of Administration:	Usually given deep IM. It may be given slow IV push
Dosage Range (Adult):	1 mg/Kg up to 25 mg IV 10-50 mg IM
Dosage Range (Pediatric):	0.5 mg to 1 mg/Kg up to 25 mg IV or IM
Supplied:	50 mg/1ml vials, ampules, and prefilled syringes
Special Considerations:	Watch for hypotension. Concurrent use with alcohol may enhance the side effects.

Dopamine
(doe'pa-meen)

Trade Name:	Dopastat, Intropin
Generic Name:	Dopamine
Classification:	Endogenous catecholamine
Actions:	Dopamine is a vasopressive agent that exhibits various

responses depending on the dose administered. Low doses (1-2 mcg/Kg/min) stimulate dopaminergic receptors which cause vasodilatation of the renal and mesenteric arteries which increase blood flow to the kidneys. Medium range doses (2-10 mcg/Kg/min) stimulate the beta receptors and increase the force of contraction of the heart to increase blood pressure. Above 10 mcg/Kg/min there is stimulation of alpha receptors in the systemic arteries (including renal and mesenteric) which cause vasoconstriction and increased peripheral vascular resistance (PVR).

Indications: Hypotension once volume losses have been re-established. Post cardiac arrest with a good heart rate (above 60) and a systolic blood pressure less than 90 mmHg. May be used to increase bradycardic heart rates refractory to atropine. TCA overdoses with hypotention.

Contraindications: Tachyarrhythmias, ventricular fibrillation, hypovolemia.

Side Effects:	Hypertension, ventricular tachyarrhythmias. Dopamine may cause nausea and vomiting.
Route of Administration:	IV infusion
Dosage Range (Adult):	2-20 mcg/Kg/minute (Dopaminergic: 1-2 mcg/kg/min; Beta: 2-10 mcg/Kg/min; Alpha: over 10 mcg/Kg/min). Generally, dopamine is started at 2-5 mcg/Kg/min (30 gtts/min) and titrated to a systolic blood pressure of 90 or 100. (See Adult Dopamine Infusion Chart.)
Drip Mixture (Adult):	400 mg in 500 ml NS or 200 mg in 250 ml to give 800 mcg/ml; 400 mg in 250 ml to give 1600 mcg/ml
Dosage Range (Pediatric):	2-20 mcg/Kg/minute. Starting dose: 5-10 mcg/Kg/min. Drip Mixture: Add 100 mg (2.5 ml of a 40 mg/ml solution) dopamine into 250 ml NS or 200 mg (5 ml of a 40 mg/ml solution) into 500 ml NS (400 mcg/ml concentiation). Using a 60 gtt/ml IV administration set, start the drip rate off at the

patient's weight in Kg which will start the infusion at 6.7 mcg/Kg/min. **(See Pediatric Dopamine Infusion Chart, pg. 24)**

Example: To start an infusion at 6.7 mcg/Kg/min for a 24 Kg child, mix 100 mg (2.5 ml of a 40 mg/ml solution) in 250 ml NS and start the infusion rate at 24 gtts/min using a 60 gtt/ml IV administration set.

$$\frac{6.7 \text{ mcg} \times \textbf{24} \text{ Kg} \times 60 \text{ gtts/ml}}{100 \text{ mg in } 250 \text{ ml NS} \ (400 \text{ mcg/ml})} = \textbf{24} \text{ gtts/ and titrate to effect}$$

Supplied:

200 mg/5 ml (40 mg/ml) or 400 mg/5 ml (80 mg/ml) pre-filled syringes and ampules

Special Considerations:

Dopamine is a very potent pressor agent. Use with caution. As with all catecholamines, dopamine should not be mixed with sodium bicarbonate.

Epinephrine 1:1,000
(ep-i-nef'ren)

Trade Name: Adrenalin

Generic Name: Epinephrine 1:1000

Classification.   Endogenous catacholamine, sympathomimetic

Actions:	Epinephrine contains both alpha and beta properties. It is both a positive chronotropic and inotropic drug as well as a potent bronchodilator.
Indications:	Acute bronchial asthma, life threatening anaphylaxis. Repeat IVP doses for cardiac arrest in pediatric patients. May be used for repeat doses for adults in cardiac arrest depending upon protocol.
Contraindications:	Tachyarrhythmias, patients with hypertension, asthmatic patients 35 years old and older (increased workload on heart can precipitate an MI)
Side Effects:	Palpitations, anxiousness, headache, tachyarrhythmias, hypertension, and vomiting
Route of Administration:	Subcutaneous, IV, ETT, IV infusion, IO
Dosage Range (Adult):	Anaphylaxis and asthma: 0.01 mg/Kg usually 0.3-0.5 mg (0.3-0.5 ml) subcutaneously
	ETT: mix 2.0 mg in 8 ml normal saline
	IV infusion: 2-10 mcg/min (start at 30 gtt/min and titrate to effect)

	Repeat doses in cardiac arrest: 5 mg IVP or 0.1 mg/Kg IVP
Drip Mixture (Adult):	1 mg in 500 ml normal saline = 2 mcg/ml concentration
Dosage Range (Pediatric):	Anaphylaxis and asthma: 0.01 ml/Kg (0.01 mg/Kg) up to 0.3 ml total dose
	Repeat dosages in cardiac arrest: 0.1 ml/Kg (0.1 mg/Kg) IVP, IO, ETT every 3 to 5 minutes
	IV infusion: 0.05-2 mcg/Kg/min (start at 0.1-0.3 mcg/Kg/min and titrate to effect).
Drip Mixture (Pediatric):	Children 2 -20 Kg: Add 3 mg (3 ml) into 250 ml NS (12 mcg/ml concentration). Using a 60 gtt/ml IV administration set starting the drip rate off at the patient's weight in Kg to administer the infusion at 0.2 mcg/kg/min. and titrate to effect.
	Children 21-40 Kg: Add 6 mg (6 ml) into 250 ml NS (24 mcg/ml concentration). Using a 60 gtt/ml IV administration set starting the drip rate off at half (1/2) the patient's weight in Kg to administer the infu-

sion at 0.2 mcg/kg/min and titrate to effect.

(See Pediatric Epinephrine Infusion Chart, pg. 25)

Example: To start an infusion off at 0.2 mcg/Kg/min for a 16 Kg child, mix 3 mg (3 ml) 1:1,000 epinephrine in 250 ml NS and start the infusion rate at 16 gtts/min using a 60 gtt/ml IV set up.

$$\frac{0.2 \text{ mcg X } \mathbf{16} \text{ Kg x 60 gtt/ml}}{\text{3 mg in 250 ml NS}} = \mathbf{16}$$

3 mg in 250 ml NS   gtts/minute
(12 mcg/ml)   and titrate
       to effect

Example: To start an infusion off at 0.2 mcg/Kg/min for a 30 Kg child, mix 6 mg (6 ml) 1:1,000 epinephrine in 250 ml NS and start the infusion rate at 15 gtts/min (half the child's weight in Kg) using a 60 gtt/ml IV set up.

$$\frac{0.2 \text{ mcg X } \mathbf{30} \text{ Kg x 60 gH/ml}}{\text{6 mg in 250 ml NS}}$$

6 mg in 250 ml NS
(24 mcg/ml) = **15** gtts/minute
          and titrate to effect

Supplied: 1 mg/1 ml ampules, 1 mg/ml 30 ml vials

Special Considerations: Epinephrine is light sensitive. Keep out of direct sunlight.

Epinephrine 1:10,000
(ep-i-nef'ren)

Trade Name:	Adrenalin
Generic Name:	Epinephrine 1:10,000
Classification:	Endogenous catecholamine, sympathomimetic
Actions:	Epinephrine contains both alpha and beta properties. Because of these properties, epinephrine will increase the following: heart rate, peripheral vascular resistance (PVR), myocardial oxygen consumption, blood pressure and automaticity of the heart.
Indications:	Epinephrine is given to pulseless patients in ventricular fibrillation, asystole, pulseless ventricular tachycardia, pulseless electrical activity (PEA). It may also be used in severe anaphylaxis IV slow push if 1:1,000 has not worked. It is the drug of choice in pediatric bradycardias unresponsive to ventilations.
Contraindications:	None when used in the above situations
Side Effects:	Tachyarrhythmias may occur after conversion of an arrested

patient. Severe nausea/vomiting in a conscious patient if given IV push.

Route of Administration: IV, IO

Dosage Range (Adult): <u>Cardiac arrest including ventricular fibrillation, pulseless ventricular tachycardia, asystole and PEA:</u> 1.0 mg IV push repeated every 3-5 minutes.

<u>Anaphylaxis refractory to SQ 1:1,000 epinephrine</u>: 0.01 ml/Kg (0.001 mg/Kg)1:10,000 IV slow push up to 5 ml (0.5 mg).

Dosage Range (Pediatric): <u>Pulseless arrest:</u> epinephrine 1:10,000 is given as the first dose of 0.1 ml/Kg (0.01 mg/Kg) IV or IO. (1:1,000 epinephrine is used in subsequent doses.)

<u>Bradycardia:</u> 1:10,000 is given 0.1 mL/Kg (0.01 mg/Kg) every 3-5 minutes

Supplied: 1 mg/10 ml, prefilled syringes

Special Considerations: Like other catecholamines, epinephrine should not be given or mixed with sodium bicarbonate because it will be deactivated. Epinephrine is light sensitive. IV, IO doses should be followed by 20 ml saline flush.

Flumazenil
(floo-maz'een-ill)

Trade Name:	Mazicon, Romazicon
Generic Name:	Flumazenil
Classification:	Benzodiazepine antidote
Actions:	Antagonizes the CNS effects of benzodiazapines by competing with specific receptor sites. It is not effective in reversing the effects of nonbenzodiazepine agents such as narcotics. Onset of action is within 1-2 minutes.
Indications:	Management of acute benzodiazepine overdose such as diazepam (Valium) and midazolam (Versed)
Contraindications:	Benzodiazepine dependent patients may experience withdrawal symptoms after administration. Hypersensitivity to this drug. Do not use in patients suspected of tricyclic antidepressant overdoses.
Side Effects:	Dyspnea, hyperventilation, seizures, bradycardia, tachycardia, and hypertension. Patients may become agitated during reversal and may need to be restrained.

Route of Administration: IV

Dosage Range (Adult):   0.2 mg over 30 seconds. If the desired changes are not achieved in 1-2 minutes, repeat at 0.3 mg over 30 seconds to a maximum dose of 3.0 mg.

Dosage Range (Pediatric):   Not recommended

Supplied: Ampules of 5 ml and 10 ml containing 0.1 mg/ml

Special Considerations: This medication has numerous incompatibilities with other drugs. Do not repeat if the patient begins twitching, is having focal seizures, or begins jerking after first dose.

Furosemide
(fur-oh'se-mide)

Trade Name: Lasix

Generic Name: Furosemide

Classification: Diuretic

Actions: Inhibits reabsorption of sodium and chloride in the kidneys promoting rapid diuresis of excess body fluid. Lasix also causes venous vasodilation which reduces preload on the heart.

Indications:	To reverse fluid overload associated with CHF and pulmonary edema. To temporarily control hypertensive crisis in certain situations.
Contraindications:	Pregnancy, hypokalemia, hypotension, sensitivity to furosemide, electrolyte imbalances, volume depletion
Side Effects:	Immediate side effects: Hypotension if given too rapidly. Nausea and vomiting, potassium depletion, and dehydration. Use with caution with patients taking Digoxin.
Route of Administration:	Slow IV push
Dosage Range (Adult):	1 mg/Kg slow IV push
Dosage Range (Pediatric):	1 mg/Kg slow IVP (usual maximum dose 20 mg)
Supplied:	2 ml ampules containing 10 mg/ml and 10 mg/ml prefilled syringes of 100 mg/10 ml or 40 mg/4 ml
Special Considerations:	Hypokalemia may be suspected in a patient who has been on chronic diuretic therapy. Protect from light. Incompatible in the same IV line with dopamine and epinephrine. Do not mix with Valium or Benadryl.

Glucagon
(gloo'kah-gon)

Trade Name:	None
Generic Name:	Glucagon HCl
Classification:	Antihypoglycemic agent, hormone
Actions:	Causes the breakdown of glycogen stores in the liver to promote increased serum glucose levels. It is also a smooth muscle relaxant.
Indications:	Hypoglycemia; second line drug of choice after 50% Dextrose if IV access is not possible
Contraindications:	Hypersensitivity to the drug. Use with caution in patients with renal, hepatic, or cardiovascular disease.
Side Effects:	Relatively few, occasionally nausea and vomiting
Route of Administration:	IV, IM (if IV in place give 50% Dextrose). Should not be given through normal saline.
Dosage Range (Adult):	1-2 mg
Dosage Range (Pediatric):	0.03 mg/Kg up to 1 mg deep IM for a single dose
Supplied:	1 mg vial (needs to be mixed) with one ml of diluent provid-

ed. Do not mix with normal saline.

Special Considerations: Glucagon is only effective if the liver has sufficient glycogen stores. It is sometimes used for the relief of esophageal foreign body obstructions and for beta blocker medication overdoses.

Ipecac
(ip'e-kak)

Trade Name: None

Generic Name: Syrup of ipecac

Classification: Emetic

Actions: Syrup of ipecac is a local irritant to the stomach and a stimulant to the emetic area of the brain which causes vomiting. Onset of action is less than 20 minutes. 80% to 90% of people given ipecac vomit within 30 minutes.

Indications: To induce emesis to rid the stomach of certain ingested poisons and medications in the conscious patient

Contraindications: Decreased level of consciousness, absent gag reflex, pregnancy, acute MI, children under 12 years of age, caustics, strong acids or bases, petroleum products, strychnine, cyanide, and phenothiazines

Side Effects: Major side effect is aspiration of vomitus. May cause hypotension and seizures.

Route of Administration: Oral

Dosage Range (Adult): 30 ml (2 tablespoons) followed by several glasses of water

Dosage Range (Pediatric): <u>Children less than 1 year of age:</u> 5-10 ml (1-2 teaspoon) follow by as much water as possible

<u>Children 1-15 years of age:</u> 15 ml (one tablespoon) followed by several glasses of water (do not use milk or carbonated beverages)

Supplied: Bottles containing 30 ml of ipecac

Special Considerations: To help promote patient emesis, have the patient walk around or increase their activity

Isoproterenol
(eye-soe-proe-ter'e-nole)

Trade Name:	Isuprel, Isopro
Generic Name:	Isoproterenol
Classification:	Sympathomimetic, bronchodilator
Actions:	Isuprel is a pure beta agonist drug. Its actions are specific to the heart and lungs. As a beta drug, it has both positive chronotropic and inotropic properties which increase the rate and force of contraction of the heart.
Indications:	Symptomatic bradycardia unresponsive to atropine. May be used in refractory Torsades de Pointe.
Contraindications:	Used with caution with suspected AMI patient because of increased work load on the heart. Ventricular ectopic beats, ventricular tachycardia, and fibrillation.
Side Effects:	Ventricular ectopy, tachyarrhythmias, ventricular tachycardia, and fibrillation
Route of Administration:	IV infusion
Dosage Range (Adult):	2-10 mcg/min titrated to effect.

Drip Mixture (Adult):	1 mg in 500 ml NS to equal a 2 mcg/ml concentration
Dosage Range (Pediatric):	Rarely used, if at all
Supplied:	1 mg/5 ml ampules or pre-filled syringes
Special Considerations:	Isuprel is titrated to a heart rate of 60 beats per minute or until PVC's occur. Isuprel is not used as a vasopressor.

Lidocaine
(lye'doe-kane)

Trade Name:	Xylocaine
Generic Name:	Lidocaine HCl
Classification:	Antiarrhythmic, local anesthetic
Actions:	Lidocaine decreases ventricular ectopy by suppressing spontaneous depolarization of ventricular pacemaker cells and raises the fibrillation threshold level.
Indications:	Lidocaine is given to patients who are symptomatic with one or more of the following: more than 6 PVC's a minute, multi focal PVC's, R on T phenomenon, coupled or paired PVC's, runs of two or more PVC's, ventricular tachy-

cardia, and ventricular fibrillation.

Contraindications: Sensitivity to the specific drug lidocaine. Third degree heart blocks, idioventricular rhythms, sinus bradycardia with escape PVC's.

Side Effects: Early lidocaine toxicity causes drowsiness, disorientation, decreased hearing, paresthesias, muscle twitching, decreased LOC and other CNS depressive signs. Severe lidocaine toxicity causes seizures. Elderly patients (70 years or older) with impaired liver function can have toxic levels accumulate quickly. These patients, as well as those patients with known liver disease, should be given half (50%) of the normal maintenance infusion once the loading dose has been given.

Route of Administration: IV, IO, IV infusion, transtracheal (ETT)

Dosage Range (Adult): Pulseless VT or VF: 1.5 mg/Kg IV repeated 1 time every 3 to 5 minutes up to a total of 3 mg/Kg

PVC's or VT with a pulse: 1-

1.5 mg/Kg IV repeated at 0.75 mg/Kg IV every 3 to 5 minutes up to a total of 3 mg/kg <u>Maintenance infusion:</u> 2-4 mg/min. (Give half of this for patients with an acute MI, CHF, shock, age greater than 70, or those with hepatic dysfunction.)

<u>ETT:</u> 2 times the IV dose

Drip Mixture (Adult): 1 gram in 250 ml NS or 2 grams in 500 ml NS to equal a 4 mg/ml concentration

Dosage Range (Pediatric): IV, IO: 1 mg/Kg q 10-15 minutes

<u>IV infusion:</u> 20-50 mcg/Kg/min

Drip Mixture(Pediatric): Mix 300 mg into 250 ml normal saline to equal a 1200 mcg/ml concentration. Using a 60 gtt/ml IV administration set, start the infusion off at the patient's weight in Kg to administer the infusion at 20 mcg/Kg/min and titrate to effect.

(See Pediatric Lidocaine Infusion Chart, pg. 27)

Example: To start an infusion off at 20 mcg/Kg/min for a 26 Kg child, mix 300 mg of lidocaine in 250 ml NS and start the infusion rate at 26 gtts/min using a 60 gtt/ml IV set up.

$$\frac{20 \text{ mcg} \times \mathbf{26} \text{ Kg} \times 60 \text{ gtt/ml}}{300 \text{ mg in } 250 \text{ ml NS}} = \mathbf{26}$$
(1200 mcg/ml)

gtts/minute and titrate to effect

Supplied: 100 mg/5 ml (20 mg/ml) in prefilled syringes and 1 or 2 grams/20 ml prefilled syringes and ampules for adult infusion preparation

Special Considerations: All IV, IO doses should be followed by a 20 ml fluid bolus. Treat lidocaine toxic seizures with Valium.

Magnesium Sulfate

Trade Name: None

Generic Name: Magnesium sulfate

Classification: Anticonvulsant; electrolyte replacement

Actions: CNS depressant, anticonvulsant, and elevates blood magnesium levels. Causes bronchodilation.

Indications: Seizures accompanying eclampsia (toxemia of pregnancy), documented hypomagnesemia. Treatment of choice for Torsades de Pointes. Can be used in refractory ventricular fibrillation, ventricular tachycardia, and asthma.

Contraindications: Heart blocks or recent MI, patients with hypotension, patients on digitalis or other cardiac glycosides, patients with respiratory depression

Side Effects: Hypotension, respiratory and neurologic depression, hyper-magnesemia, heart blocks

Route of Administration: IV slow push, IV infusion

Dosage Range (Adult): Eclampsia: 2-4 grams diluted in 100 ml NS given IV slow push or by infusion

Torsades and refractory ventricular fibrillation and ventricular tachycardia: 1-2 grams IV slow push

Supplied: 500 mg/ml 10 ml vials

Special Considerations: Calcium chloride should be readily available as an antidote if respiratory depression occurs. Do not mix magnesium sulfate with sodium bicarbonate.

Meperidine HCl
(me-per'i-deen)

Trade Name:	Demerol
Generic Name:	Meperidine HCl
Classification:	Narcotic, analgesic
Actions:	Decreases pain response by binding with opioid receptors in the brain
Indications:	Relief of moderate to severe pain
Contraindications:	Patients on MAO inhibitors, abdominal pain, head injury, stroke, hypersensitivity to Demerol. Patient with respiratory compromise.
Side Effects:	Respiratory depression, hypotension, drowsiness, seizures
Route of Administration:	IV
Dosage Range (Adult):	1mg/Kg IV titrated to effect
Dosage Range (Pediatric):	IV, IO: 1 mg/Kg up to 50 mg slow IV push
Supplied:	50 mg/ml ampules and vials
Special Considerations:	Side effects can be reversed with naloxone (Narcan)

Methylprednisolone

(meth-ill-pred-niss'oh-lone)

Trade Name:	Solu-medrol
Generic Name:	Methylprednisolone
Classification:	Corticosteroid, anti-inflammatory agent
Actions:	Strengthens cell membrane walls which decreases cell/capillary membrane permeability reducing edema. Inhibits cells from releasing vasodilating agents during allergic reactions.
Indications:	Acute anaphylactic reactions, acute asthma, cerebral edema, and acute spinal cord damage
Contraindications:	None in the prehospital setting other than known hypersensitivity to the drug
Side Effects:	None with single dose use
Route of Administration:	IV
Dosage Range (Adult):	Anaphylactic shock, acute asthma: 2 mg/Kg or 125 mg doses

Spinal cord injury: 30 mg/Kg loading dose |
| **Dosage Range (Pediatric):** | Anaphylactic shock, acute asthma: 1-2 mg/Kg doses

Spinal cord injury: 30 mg/Kg |

loading dose

Supplied: Vials for injection containing 125 mg and 500 mg

Midazolam
(mye-da'-zoe-lam)

Trade Name: Versed

Generic Name: Midazolam

Classification: Benzodiazepine

Actions: Versed is a short acting benzo-diazepine which produces CNS depression with some amnectic effects. It easily crosses the blood brain barrier to cause deep sedation. It is 3 to 4 times as potent as Valium. It has no analgesic effects.

Indications: Generalized seizures; status epilepticus; sedation prior to cardioversion

Contraindications: Known hypersensitivity to this drug. Pregnancy, patients in shock or coma, known ETOH ingestion, and respiratory depression. Use with caution in patients with respiratory diseases such as COPD and CHF.

Side Effects: Respiratory depression and/or arrest is possible if given rapid

	IVP. Hypotension and tachycardia, especially in older adults.
Route of Administration:	Slow IV push, deep IM
Dosage Range (Adult):	Slow IV: 0.5 mg up to 5 mg titrated to effect
	Deep IM: 5 mg. Consider lower doses for patients with respiratory diseases or patients older than 60.
Dosage Range (Pediatric):	Slow IV, IO, or deep IM 0.1-0.3 mg/Kg up to 5 mg.
Supplied:	2-10 ml vials of 5-50 mg and 2 ml prefilled syringes containing 10 mg (5 mg/ml)
Special Considerations:	Patients should be placed on a monitor and watched closely for adverse effects during the administration of Versed. Watch for possible respiratory depression and arrest. To reverse the side effects of Versed, have flumazenil (Mazicon) available.

Morphine Sulfate
(Mor' feen súl-fate)

Trade Name:	Duramorph, Infumorph
Generic Name:	Morphine sulfate, MS

Classification:	Narcotic, analgesic
Actions:	Morphine is a powerful pain killer. It is also an arterial and venodilator which pools blood and decreases both preload and afterload of the heart. This decreases work load on the heart which decreases myocardial oxygen demand. It is a CNS depressant which helps to alleviate anxiety.
Indications:	Chest pain unrelieved by nitroglycerin. Pulmonary edema. Severe (non-cardiac) pain.
Contraindications:	Hypotension, head injury, abdominal injury or pain
Side Effects:	Respiratory depression, hypotension, nausea, and vomiting
Route of Administration:	IV slow push, IM
Dosage Range (Adult):	Small increments of 1-3 mg every 5-30 minutes. Use lower doses in the elderly.
Dosage Range (Pediatric):	0.05-0.1 mg/Kg slow IV push
Supplied:	Prefilled syringes containing 10 mg/1 mL
Special Considerations:	Narcan should be readily available to reverse the effects of morphine

Naloxone HCl

(nal-ox' own)

Trade Name:	Narcan
Generic Name:	Naloxone HCl
Classification:	Narcotic (opiate) antagonist
Actions:	Specific antidote for narcotic agents. Effective in counteracting the effects of an overdose from any of these agents by binding with narcotic receptor sites.
Indications:	Narcotic overdoses or coma of unknown origin
Contraindications:	Known hypersensitivity to the drug
Side Effects:	May precipitate acute narcotic withdrawal syndrome; may cause cardiac dysrhythmias, vomiting
Route of Administration:	IV, IM, SC, IO, or ETT
Dosage Range (Adult):	<u>IV, IM, IO:</u> 2.0 mg repeated every 2-3 minutes as necessary up to a total of 10 mg <u>ETT:</u> 4 mg added to NS for a total volume of 10 ml in a syringe
Dosage Range (Pediatric):	<u>IV, IO</u> 0.1 mg/Kg up to 2 mg. May repeat in 5 minutes. ETT: 2-3 times the IV dose

Supplied: Vials of 2 mg/1 ml; prefilled syringes of 2 mg/5 ml

Special Considerations: Narcan should be given slow IVP. The patient should be restrained, if possible, prior to administration. Monitor respirations for a guide as to its effectiveness. Narcan may have a shorter half life than the narcotic and the patient may need repeat doses. Large doses may be required to reverse the effects of Darvon (Darvocet).

Narcan will reverse the effects of the following drugs:

1. Codeine
2. Darvon
3. Demerol
4. Dilaudid
5. Fentanyl
6. Heroin
7. Methadone
8. Morphine
9. Nubain
10. Paregoric
11. Percodan
12. Stadol
13. Talwin

Nitroglycerin
(nye-troe-gli'ser-in)

Trade Name: Sublingual: Nitrostat, Nitrolingual spray

IV: Nitro-bid, Nitrol, Nitrostat

Generic Name: Nitroglycerin

Classification: Antianginal, nitrate

Actions:	Nitroglycerin relaxes smooth muscle of coronary arteries and veins. This reduces preload on the heart and increases perfusion to ischemic myocardial tissue.
Indications:	Chest pain due to angina pectoris; hypertensive crisis; CHF and pulmonary edema
Contraindications:	Increased intracranial pressure, hypotension (systolic less than 90 mmHg)
Side Effects:	Headache, hypotension, syncope
Route of Administration:	Sublingual tablets, spray; IV infusion
Dosage Range (Adult):	<u>Tablets:</u> 0.3 mg (1/200 gr) or 0.4 mg (1/150 gr) sublingual every 5 minutes up to three tablets have been given or complete relief

<u>Spray:</u> 1 sublingual spray every 5 minutes up to 3 sprays or complete relief

IV Infusion: 5-10 mcg/min (3-6 gtts/min using a 60 gtt/ml IV administration set) slowly titrating to pain relief or until hypotension ensues

(See Adult Nitroglycerin Infusion Chart, pg. 15)

Drip Mixture:	5 ml (25 mg) in 250 ml NS to equal a 100 mcg/ml concentration
Supplied:	0.3 mg (1/200 gr) or 0.4 mg (1/150 gr) tablets in bottles containing 30 or 100 tablets
	Nitrolingual spray is a metered dose of 0.4 mg per spray
	5 ml ampules containing 5 mg/ml (25 mg)
Special Considerations:	Once bottle is open, nitroglycerin expires rapidly. Be sure that nitro is not out-of-date or has lost its effectiveness. Nitro is light sensitive. <u>Remember to take BP before and after administration of this drug!</u> Patients may have a nitro patch on which may be the cause of hypotension/syncopal episodes. Remove the patch if you are going to defibrillate. Make sure you do not get any nitro paste on yourself.

Nitrous Oxide

Trade Name:	Nitronox
Generic Name:	Nitrous oxide, N_2O
Classification:	Analgesic (anesthetic gas)
Actions:	Nitronox is a 50:50 mixture of

nitrous oxide and oxygen that is inhaled and absorbed into the blood stream to give potent analgesic effects.

Indications: Moderate to severe pain due to AMI, musculoskleletal trauma, burns, or kidney stones

Contraindications: Head injury, increased intracranial pressure, shock, abdominal injuries, bowel obstructions, COPD or other respiratory diseases. Patients with altered mental status or those who are unable to self-administer the gas.

Side Effects: Nausea and vomiting are possible. If it is believed the patient has taken too much, remove the mask and administer straight oxygen. Never secure the mask to the patient's face!

Route of Administration: Self-inhalation by the patient only

Dosage Range (Adult): Self-administration by mask. Once patient has had enough and the pain is relieved, the patient will drop the mask and begin to breathe room air.

Dosage Range (Pediatric): Same as adult

Supplied: Generally comes in a pack or case containing one E cylinder (blue) of nitrous oxide and one E cylinder (green) of oxygen. A special regulator mixes the gases to the right concentration.

Special Considerations: When using nitrous oxide in a closed space (back of the unit) have the windows open. Gas leak from the patient mask seal may overcome the paramedic and the driver.

Oxygen
(o´x-a-gin)

Trade Name: None

Generic Name: Oxygen

Classification: Medical gas

Actions: Oxygen is necessary for all normal cellular functions. It makes up for 21% of atmospheric air. It raises blood oxygen tension and hemoglobin saturation levels.

Indications: All patients who are hypoxic. Any physiologic condition where increased oxygen delivery will be beneficial.

Contraindications: None, if indicated

Side Effects:	None, if used appropriately
Route of Administration:	Multiple delivery methods are available
	(See the supplemental oxygen delivery chart, pg. 131)
Dosage Range (Adult):	24 to 100% depending on the liter flow and the method of delivery
Dosage Range (Pediatric):	24 to 100% depending on the liter flow and the method of delivery
Supplied:	In the prehospital setting, oxygen is contained in various sizes of green cylinders
Special Considerations:	In the prehospital setting, oxygen should never be withheld. In certain medical conditions (AMI, stroke, COPD), the delivery of oxygen should be initially started at a low level and then titrated up to meet the demands of the patient and their physiologic needs.

Oxytocin
(ox-a-toe'sin)

Trade Name:	Pitocin
Generic Name:	Oxytocin
Classification:	Hormone

Actions:	Causes uterine contraction, lactation, slows postpartum bleeding
Indications:	Control of postpartum vaginal hemorrhage after the delivery of infant(s) and placenta
Contraindications:	History of a previous cesarean section (c-section), prior to delivery of multiple babies or prior to the delivery of the placenta
Side Effects:	Anaphylaxis, cardiac arrhythmias, uterine rupture
Route of Administration:	IV infusion
Dosage Range (Adult):	Infusion of 10 units in 500 ml NS starting at 20-40 milliunits per minute titrated to effect
Supplied:	10 units/ml in 1 mL ampules
Drip Mixture:	10 units (l ml) in 500 ml NS = 20 milliunits/ml
Special Considerations:	Do not use concurrently with other vasopressors.

Procainamide
(proe-ka´ne-amide)

Trade Name:	Pronestyl, Procan, Promine
Generic Name:	Procainamide HCl
Classification:	Antiarrhythmic

Actions:	Same actions as for lidocaine and bretylium. An added advantage of procainamide, unlike lidocaine and bretylium, is that it has some anti-arrhythmic effects on supraventricular rhythms and atrial ectopic pacemakers.
Indications:	PVC's and ventricular tachycardia refractory to lidocaine. SVT not responding to adenosine.
Contraindications:	Heart blocks
Side Effects:	Hypotension, dizziness, bradycardia, Torsades de Pointes
Route of Administration:	Slow IV loading infusion, IV maintenance infusion
Dosage Range (Adult):	<u>IV loading infusion:</u> 20 mg/min by adding 1 gram (1 g/10 ml) to 40 ml NS to equal 20 mg/ml. Infuse using a 60 gtt/ml IV administration set at 60 gtts/min. Infuse the procainamide until either the arrhythmia is suppressed, hypotension develops, the QRS complex widens by 50%, or a total of 17 mg/kg has been given. <u>Maintenance infusion</u>: 1-4 mg/min.

Drip Mixture (Adult):	1 gram in 500 ml NS to equal a 2 mg/ml concentration
Dosage Range (Pediatric):	Rare to use
Supplied:	10 ml vials of 1 gram (100 mg/ml), or 2 ml vials of 1 gram (500 mg/ml)
Special Considerations:	This drug takes a long time to completely administer.

Prochlorperazine
(proe-klor-per'a-zeen)

Trade Name:	Compazine
Generic Name:	Prochlorperazine
Classification:	Antiemetic, tranquilizer, phenothiazine
Actions:	Blocks the neurotransmitter dopamine to depress various areas of the CNS including wakefulness, temperature regulation, and emesis control
Indications:	Control of nausea and vomiting from a variety of causes
Contraindications:	Known hypersensitivity to Compazine, comatose or stuporous patients. Alcohol ingestions.
Side Effects:	Sedation, hypotension, seizures, cardiovascular collapse. Dystonic muscle spasms

to neck and back causing an inability to control the airway. Dystonic reaction may be controlled with IV Benadryl.

Route of Administration: Slow IV over 2-5 minutes, IM

Dosage Range (Adult): <u>IV:</u> 5-10 mg watching for hypotension. In older patients consider half doses. 5-10 mg deep IM.

Supplied: 5 mg/ml in 2 ml vials

Special Considerations: Avoid skin contact when handling Compazine. It will cause contact dermatitis. Treat seizures with Valium. Compazine is incompatible with Versed.

Proparacaine
(pro-pár-a'kane)

Trade Name: Alcaine, Ophthaine

Generic Name: Proparacaine

Classification: Topical eye anesthetic

Actions: Blocks pain receptors. Onset of action is 30-60 seconds and lasts for 15 minutes up to 1-2 hours.

Indications: Relief of eye pain due to a foreign body, corneal abrasions, flash burns, and irritating chemicals. To allow for patient cooperation during irrigation of the eyes.

Contraindications:	Hypersensitivity to proparacaine, ruptured globe
Side Effects:	Stinging, lacrimation, photophobia
Route of Administration:	Drop application
Dosage Range (Adult):	1-2 drops in the affected eye
Supplied:	0.5% proparacaine in 15 ml of solution
Special Considerations:	The drops will sting at first but will provide pain relief in a few seconds. Do not give the patient the remaining solution for their own use. Continual application of proparacaine will inhibit healing.

Sodium Bicarbonate

Trade Name:	None
Generic Name:	Sodium bicarbonate
Classification:	Alkalinizing agent, electrolye replacement
Actions:	Neutralizes excess acid in the blood and interstitial fluid. Returns blood to a normal physiologic pH by increasing the availability of the bicarbonate ion.
Indications:	Pre-existing metabolic acidosis associated with cardiac arrest,

shock, and DKA.
Hyperkalemia. To promote the excretion of some types of barbiturate and salicylate overdoses. Tricyclic anti-depressant overdose and crush injuries.

Contraindications: Hypokalemia. Conditions in which a patient cannot handle an increased salt load, such as CHF or renal failure. Metabolic alkalosis.

Side Effects: Increases intravascular volume. Lowers serum potassium. Raises the arterial carbon dioxide levels. Inactivates catecholamines. Metabolic alkalosis. Tissue necrosis if infiltrated at the IV site.

Route of Administration: IV, IV infusion

Dosage Range (Adult): IV: 1 mEq/Kg repeating half (1/2) the initial dose every 10 minutes

Crush injuries: add 50 ml (50 mEq) in 1000 ml NS or 0.45% NS and infuse

Dosage Range (Pediatric): 1 year and older: 1 mEq/Kg IV (can repeat every 10 minutes) using a 8.4% solution

Newborn to 1 year old: 1-2 mEq/Kg IV (can repeat every

10 minutes) using a 4.2% solution

To make a 4.2% solution, squirt out 25 ml from an 8.4% solution and replace it with 25 ml sterile H_2O

Supplied: Prefilled syringes of 50 ml containing 1 mEq/ml (8.4%)

Special Considerations: Flush the IV line well when using sodium bicarbonate before or after epinephrine or calcium chloride. During cardiac arrest, do not over use. Metabolic alkalosis is difficult to counteract in the field. IVP doses should be followed by a 20 ml saline flush.

Tetracaine HCl
(tét-ra kane)

Trade Name: Pontocaine

Generic Name: Tetracaine HCl

Classification: Topical eye anesthetic

Actions: Blocks pain receptors. Onset of action is 30-60 seconds and lasts 15 minutes up to 1-2 hours.

Indications: Relief of eye pain due to a foreign body, corneal abrasions, flash burns, and irritating chemicals. To allow for patient cooperation during irrigation of the eyes.

Contraindications: Hypersensitivity to tetracaine, ruptured globe

Side Effects: Stinging, lacrimation, photophobia

Route of Administration: Drop application

Dosage Range (Adult): 1-2 drops in the affected eye

Supplied: 0.5% tetracaine in 15 ml of solution

Special Considerations: The drops will sting at first but will provide pain relief in a few seconds. Do not give the patient the remaining solution for their own use. Continual application of tetracaine will inhibit healing.

Thiamine
(thy'a-men)

Trade Name: Betalin, Biamine

Generic Name: Thiamine (vitamin B_1)

Classification: Water soluble vitamin

Actions: Needed for normal metabolism of carbohydrates (glucose)

Indications: Treatment of thiamine deficiency (beriberi). Typically given along with D50 for comas of unknown origin in suspected alcoholics.

Contraindications:	Hypersensitivity
Side Effects:	Severe anaphylaxis in hypersensitive patients. Heart failure.
Route of Administration:	IV
Dosage Range (Adult):	100 mg IV slow push
Supplied:	5 ml and 10 ml (100 mg/ml) vials and syringes
Special Considerations:	Commonly given to alcoholics along with D50 to prevent Wernicke's encephalopathy.

Verapamil
(ver-ap'a-mill)

Trade Name:	Calan, Isoptin
Generic Name:	Verapamil
Classification:	Calcium ion antagonist (calcium channel blocker)
Actions:	Verapamil blocks the entry of calcium into both cardiac and smooth muscle causing prolonged refractory periods. Verapamil is useful in controlling re-entry arrhythmias such as atrial fibrillation and atrial flutter. With its vasodilating

properties, verapamil will increase coronary artery perfusion, decrease afterload, and cause a decrease in blood pressure. Verapamil is a negative inotropic drug, which decreases myocardial oxygen consumption.

Indications: Verapamil is a second line drug after adenosine for narrow complex supraventricular tachycardias with a stable blood pressure that does not require cardioversion. In the absence of Wolff-Parkinson White syndrome (WPW), it is the drug of choice for symptomatic atrial fibrillation and atrial flutter with rapid ventricular response.

Contraindications: Verapamil should be avoided in patients taking beta blockers. It should not be given to patients with Wolff-Parkinson White syndrome (WPW), with known Sick Sinus syndrome, any wide complex tachycardia, heart failure, or heart blocks.

Side Effects: Hypotension, possible asystole, ventricular fibrillation

Route of Administration: IV slow push over 1-3 minutes (onset of action may take 3-5 minutes).

Dosage Range (Adult): 2.5 to 5 mg initial dose. May repeat at 5-10 mg every 15-30 minutes. Patients over 70 years of age should receive smaller doses (2-4 mg) over a longer period of time (3-4 minutes).

Supplied: 5 mg/2 ml (2.5 mg/ml) ampules and prefilled syringes

Special Considerations: Continually monitor the patient's blood pressure for signs of hypotension before, during, and after administration. Avoid using in conjunction with sodium bicarbonate or patients taking theophylline.

Overdose: Calcium chloride may be useful in reversing the hypotensive side effects of a verapamil overdose.

Common Prescription Medications and Their Uses

Brand to Generic

Brand Name	Generic Name	Type of Drug
Accupril	quinapril HCl	Cardiac drug
Adalat	nifedipine	Cardiac drug
Advil	ibuprofen	Non steroidal anti-inflammatory agent
Aldactazide	hydrochlorothiazide	Diuretic
Allegra	fexofenadine HCl	Antihistamine drug
Altace	ramipril	Cardiac drug
Ambien	zolpiden tartrate	Sedative/hypnotic
Amoxil	amoxicillin trihydrate	Antibiotic
Antispas	dicycolmine HCl	GI - antispasmodic
Apresoline	hydralazine HCl	Antihypertensive
Ativan	lorazepam	Sedative/hypnotic (benzodiazepine)
Atrovent	ipratropium bromide	Anticholinergic agent
Augmentin	amoxicillin & potassium clavulanate	Antibiotic
Axid	nizatidine	GI drug (H_2 antagonist)
Azmacort	triamcinolone acetonide	Corticosteroid
Bactrim	trimethoprim & sulfa	Antibiotic
Bactroban	mupirocin	Antibiotic
Bemote	dicycolmine HCl	GI - antispasmodic
Bentyl	dicycolmine HCl	GI - antispasmodic
Biaxin	clarithromycin	Antibiotic

Brand Name	Generic Name	Type of Drug
Bumex	bumetanide	Diuretic
Buspar	buspirone	Sedative/hypnotic
Calan	verapamil HCl	Cardiac drug
Capoten	captopril	Cardiac drug
Cardizem	diltiazem HCl	Cardiac drug
Cardura	doxazosin mesylate	Antihypertensive
Catapres	clonidine HCl	Antihypertensive
Ceclor	cefaclor	Antibiotic
Ceftin	cefuroxime	Antibiotic
Cefzil	cefprozil	Antibiotic
Cipro	ciprofloxacin	Antibiotic
Claritin	loratadine	Antihistamine
Coumadin	warfarin sodium	Anticoagulant
Cozaar	losartan	Antihypertensive
Darvocet-N	propoxyphene napsylate	Opiate agonist, analgesic
Daypro	oxaprozin	Nonsteroid anti-inflammatory agent
Deltasone	prednisone	Corticosteroid
Depakote	divalproex sodium	Anticonvulsant
Depo-Provera	medroxyprogesterone acetate	Birth control
Desogen	none	Birth control
Desyrel	trazodone HCl	Antidepressant
Diabeta	glyburide	Oral hypoglycemic agent

Brand Name	Generic Name	Type of Drug
Diflucan	fluconazole	Antifungal antibiotic
Dilacor XR	diltiazem HCl	Cardiac drug
Dilantin	phenytoin	Anticonvulsant
Doryx	doxycycline hyclate	Antibiotic
Doxy	doxycycline hyclate	Antibiotic
Doxychel	doxycycline hyclate	Antibiotic
Dyazide	triamterene & HCTZ	Diuretic
Effexor	venlafaxine	Antidepressant
Elavil	amitriptyline HCl	Antidepressant
Elocon	mometasone furoate	Anti-inflammatory agent
Endep	amitriptyline HCl	Antidepressant
Ery-Tab	erythromycin	Antibiotic
Esidrex	hydrochlorothiazide	Diuretic
Estrace	estradiol	Estrogen
Estraderm	estradiol patch	Estrogen
Fastin	phentermine HCl	Anorexiant
Fioricet	butalbital, caffeine, APAP	Analgesic
Flexeril	cyclobenzaprine HCl	Skeletal muscle relaxant
Flonase	fluticasone	Anti-inflammatory agent
Floxin	ofloxacin	Antibiotic
Fosamax	alendronate sodium	Reabsorption inhibitor (bone)

Brand Name	Generic Name	Type of Drug
Glucophage	metformin hydrochloride	Oral hypoglycemic agent
Glucotrol XL	glipizide	Oral hypoglycemic agent
Glynase	glyburide	Oral hypoglycemic agent
Guaifenesin	robitussin, humibid	Expectorant
Humulin 70/30	none	Insulin
Hydrodiuril	hydrochlorothiazide	Diuretic
Hydropres	hydrochlorothiazide	Diuretic
Hytrin	terazosin	Antihypertensive
Imdur	isosorbide mononitrate	Vasodilating agent (oral nitrate)
Imitrex	sumatriptan succinate	Migraine analgesic
Isoptin	verapamil HCl	Cardiac drug
K-Dur	potassium chloride	Potassium supplement
K-LOA	potassium chloride	Potassium supplement
K-Lor	potassium chloride	Potassium supplement
K-Lyte/CL	potassium chloride	Potassium supplement
K-Tab	potassium chloride	Potassium supplement
Keflex	cephalexin monohydrate	Antibiotic
Klonopin	clonazepam	Benzodiazepine (anticonvulsant)
Klor-Con	potassium chloride	Potassium supplement
Klorvess	potassium chloride	Potassium supplement

Brand Name	Generic Name	Type of Drug
Lamisil	terbinafine HCl	Antifungal
Lanoxin	digoxin	Cardiac drug
Lasix	furosemide	Diuretic
Lescol	fluvastatine Sodium	Lipid lowering drug
Librax	clidinium & chlordiazepoxide	GI antispasmodic
Lidox	clidinium & chlordiazepoxide	GI antispasmodic
Lipitor	atorvastatin	Lipid lowering drug
LO/OVRAL-28	none	Birth control
Lodine	etodolac	Nonsteroidal anti-inflammatory agent
Loestrin-FE 1.5/30	none	Birth control
Loestrin-FE 1/20-2	none	Birth control
Lopid	gemfibrozil	Lipid lowering drug
Lopressor	metroprolol	Cardiac drug
Lorabid	loracarbef	Antibiotic
Lotensin	benazepril HCl	Lipid lowering drug
Lotrisone	clotrimazole & betamethasone dipropionate	Anti-fungal agent
Lozol	indapamide	Antihypertensive
Macrobid	nitrofurantoin	Antibiotic
Maxzide	triamterent & HCTZ	Diuretic
Medrol	methylprednisolone	Corticosteroid
Meticorten	prednisone	Corticosteroid

Brand Name	Generic Name	Type of Drug
Mevacor	lovastatin	Lipid lowering drug
Micro-K	potassium chloride	Potassium supplement
Micronase	glyburide	Oral hypoglycemic agent
Monodox	doxycycline hyclate	Antibiotic
Motrin	ibuprofen	Nonsteroidal anti-inflammatory agent
Naprosyn	naproxen	Nonsteroidal anti-inflammatory agent
Neosporin	neomycin	Antibiotic
Neurontin	gabapentin	Anticonvulsant
Nitro-Dur	nitroglycerin	Vasodilating agent
Nitrostat	nitroglycerin	Vasodilating agent
Nolvadex	tamoxifen citrate	Antineoplastic hormone
Norflex	orphenadrine citrate	Skeletal muscle relaxant
Norvasc	amlodipine besylate	Antihypertensive
Nuprin	ibuprofen	Nonsteroidal anti-inflammatory agent
Orasone	prednisone	Corticosteroid
Oretic	hydrochlorothiazide	Diuretic
Ortho-Cept-28	none	Birth control
Ortho-Cyclen-28	none	Birth control
Ortho-NOV 28	none	Birth control
Ortho-Tri-CY 28	none	Birth control

Brand Name	Generic Name	Type of Drug
Paxil	paroxetine HCl	Antidepressant
Pepcid	famotidine	GI drug (H_2 antagonist)
Percocert	oxycodone & APAP	Opiate agonist, analgesic
Percodan	oxycodone with ASA	Opiate agonist, analgesic
Persantine	dipyridamole	Platelet aggregation inhibitor
Phenergan	promethazine HCl	Antihistamine/antiemetic
Pravachol	pravastatine sodium	Lipid lowering drug
Precose	acarbose	Oral hypoglycemic agent
Premarin	none	Hormone/estrogen
Prempro	none	Hormone/estrogen & progesterone
Prilosec	omeprazole	GI drug (H_2 antagonist)
Prinivil	lisinopril	Cardiac drug
Procardia	nifedipine	Cardiac drug
Propulsid	cisapride	GI motility drug
Proventil	albuterol	Bronchodilator
Provera	medroxy progesterone acetate	Birth control
Prozac	fluoxetine HCl	Antidepressant
Relafen	nabumetone	Nonsteroidal anti-inflammatory agent
Restoril	temazepam	Sedative/hypnotic (benzodiazepine)
Risperdal	resperidone	Antipsycotic drug
Ritalin	methylphenidate HCl	CNS stimulant

Brand Name	Generic Name	Type of Drug
Roxicet	oxycodone HCl & APAP	Opiate agonist, analgesic
Rufen	ibuprofen	Nonsteroidal anti-inflammatory agent
Serevent	salmeterol	Bronchodilator
Serzone	nefazodone HCl	Antidepressant
Soma	carisoprodol	Skeletal muscle relaxant
Synthroid	levothyroxine sodium	Thyroid agent
Tagamet	cimetidine	GI drug (H_2 antagonist)
Tegretol	carbamazapine	Anticonvulsant
Tenoretic	atenolol & chlorthalidone	Cardiac drug
Tenormin	atenolol	Cardiac drug
Ticlid	ticlopidine HCl	Platelet aggregation inhibitor
Timolide	hydrochlorothiazide	Diuretic
Timoptic-XE	timolol muleate	Antiglaucoma
Tobradex	tobramycin & dexamethasone	Anti-inflammatory/antibiotic
Toprol-XL	metroprolol succinate	Cardiac drug
Trental	pentoxifylline	Hemorheologic agent
Tri-Levlen 28	none	Birth control
Trimox	amoxicillin trihydrate	Antibiotic
Tripphasil 28	none	Birth control
Trusopt	dorzolamide hydrochloride	Antiglaucoma
Tylenol	acetaminophen	Analgesic

Brand Name	Generic Name	Type of Drug
Ultracef	cefaclor	Antibiotic
Ultram	tramadol HCl	Opiate agonist, analgesic
Valium	diazepam	Sedative/hypnotic (benzodiazepine)
Vancenase	beclomethasone dipropionate	Anti-inflammatory agent
Vanceril	beclomethazone dipropionate	Anti-inflammatory agent
Vascor	bepridil	Antianginal
Vasotec	enalapril maleate	Cardiac drug
Veetids	penicillin v potassium	Antibiotic
Venolin	albuterol	Bronchodilator
Vibramycin	doxycycline hyclate	Antibiotic
Vicodin	hydrocodone with APAP	Opiate agonist, analgesic
Vistaril	hydroxyzine pamoate	Antihistamine/sedative
Wellbutrin	bupropion HCl	Antidepressant
Xalatan	latanoprost	Antiglaucoma
Xanax	alprazolam	Sedative/hypnotic (benzodiazepine)
Zantac	ranitidine	GI drug (H_2 antagonist)
Zarontin	ethosuximide	Anticonvulsant

Brand Name	Generic Name	Type of Drug
Zebrax	chlordiazepoxide & clidinium	GI antispasmodic
Zestoretic	hydrochlorothiazide	Antihypertensive
Zestril	lisinopril	Cardiac drug
Ziac	bisoprolol fumarate & HCTZ	Antihypertensive
Zithromax	azithromycin Dihydrate	Antibiotic
Zocor	simvastatine	Lipid lowering drug
Zoloft	sertraline HCl	Antidepressant
Zovirax	acyclovir	Antiviral
Zyloprim	allopurinol	Cardiac drug
Zyrtec	cetirizine HCl	Antihistamine

Generic to Brand

Generic Name	Brand Name	Type of Drug
acarbose	Precose	Oral hypoglycemic agent
acetaminophen	Tylenol	Analgesic
acyclovir	Zovirax	Antiviral
albuterol	Proventil, Venolin	Bronchodilator
alendronate sodium	Fosamax	Reabsorption inhibitor (bone)
allopurinol	Zyloprim	Cardiac drug
alprazolam	Xanax	Sedative/hypnotic benzodiazepine
amitriptyline HCl	Elavil, Endep	Antidepressant
amlodipine besylate	Norvasc	Antihypertensive
amoxicillin & potassium clavulanate	Augmentin	Antibiotic
amoxicillin trihydrate	Amoxil, Trimox	Antibiotic
atenolol	Tenormin	Cardiac drug
atenolol & chlorthalidone	Tenoretic	Cardiac drug
atorvastatin	Lipitor	Lipid lowering drug
azithromycin dihydrate	Zithromax	Antibiotic

beclomethasone dipropionate	Vancenase, Vanceril	Anti-inflammatory agent
benazepril HCl	Lotensin	Lipid lowering drug
bepridil	Vascor	Antianginal
bisoprolol fumarate & HCTZ	Ziac	Antihypertensive
bumetanide	Bumex	Diuretic

Generic Name	Brand Name	Type of Drug
bupropion HCl	Willbutrin	Antidepressant
buspirone	Buspar	Sedative/hypnotic
butalbital, caffeine, APAP	Fioricet	Analgesic
captopril	Capoten	Cardiac drug
carbamazapine	Tegretol	Anticonvulsant
carisoprodol	Soma	Skeletal muscle relaxant
cefaclor	Ceclor, Ultracef	Antibiotic
cefprozil	Cefzil	Antibiotic
cefuroxime	Ceftin	Antibiotic
cephalexin monohydrate	Keflex	Antibiotic
cetirizine HCl	Zyrtec	Antihistamine
chlordiazepoxide & clidinium	Zebrax	GI antispasmodic
cimetidine	Tagamet	GI drug (H_2 antagonist)
ciprofloxacin	Cipro	Antibiotic
cisapride	Propulsid	GI motility drug
clarithromycin	Biaxin	Antibiotic
clidinium & chlordiazepoxide	Librax, Lidox	GI antispasmodic
clonazepam	Klonopin	Benzodiazepine (anticonvulsant)
clonidine HCl	Catapres	Antihypertensive
clotrimazole & betamethasone dipropionate	Lotrisone	Anti-fungal agent
cyclobenzaprine HCl	Flexeril	Skeletal muscle relaxant

Generic Name	Brand Name	Type of Drug
diazepam	Valium	Sedative/hypnotic (benzodiazepine)
dicycolmine HCl	Antispas, Bemote, Bentyl	GI antispasmodic
digoxin	Lanoxin	Cardiac drug
diltiazem HCl	Cardizem, Dilacor XR	Cardiac drug
dipyridamole	Persantine	Platelet aggregation inhibitor
divalproex sodium	Depakote	Anticonvulsant
dorzolamide hydrochloride	Trusopt	Antiglaucoma
doxazosin mesylate	Cardura	Antihypertensive
doxycycline hyclate	Doryx, Doxy Doxychel, Monodox Vibramycin	Antibiotic
enalapril maleate	Vasotec	Cardiac drug
erythromycin	Ery-Tab	Antibiotic
estradiol	Estrace	Estrogen
estradiol patch	Estraderm	Estrogen
ethosuximide	Zarontin	Anticonvulsant
etodolac	Lodine	Nonsteroidal anti-inflammatory agent
famotidine	Pepcid	GI drug (H_2 antagonist)
fexofenadine HCl	Allegra	Antihistamine drug
fluconazole	Diflucan	Antifungal antibiotic
fluoxetine HCl	Prozac	Antidepressant
fluticasone	Flonase	Anti-inflammatory agent
fluvastatine Sodium	Lescol	Lipid lowering drug
furosemide	Lasix	Diuretic

Generic Name	Brand Name	Type of Drug
gabapentin	Neurontin	Anticonvulsant
gemfibrozil	Lopid	Lipid lowering drug
glipizide	Glucotrol XL	Oral hypoglycemic agent
glyburide	Diabeta, Glynase, Micronase	Oral hypoglycemic agent
hydralazine HCl	Apresoline	Antihypertensive
hydrochlorothiazide	Zestoretic	Antihypertensive
hydrochlorothiazide	Aldactazide, Esidrex, Hydrodiuril, Hydropres, Oretic, Timolide	Diuretic
hydrocodone with APAP	Vicodin	Opiate agonist, analgesic
hydroxyzine pamoate	Vistaril	Antihistamine/sedative
ibuprofen	Advil, Motrin, Nuprin, Rufen	Nonsteroidal anti-inflammatory agent
indapamide	Lozol	Antihypertensive
ipratropium bromide	Atrovent	Anticholinergic agent
isosorbide mononitrate	Imdur	Vasodilating agent (oral nitrate)
latanoprost	Xalatan	Antiglaucoma
levothyroxine sodium	Synthroid	Thyroid agent
lisinopril	Prinivil	Cardiac drug
lisinopril	Zestril	Cardiac drug
loracarbef	Lorabid	Antibiotic

Generic Name	Brand Name	Type of Drug
loratadine	Claritin	Antihistamine
lorazepam	Ativan	(Benzodiazepine) sedative/hypnotic
losartan	Cozaar	Antihypertensive
lovastatin	Mevacor	Lipid lowering drug
medroxyprogesterone acetate	Depo-Provera	Birth control
medroxyprogesterone acetate	Provera	Birth control
metformin hydrochloride	Glucophage	Oral hypoglycemic agent
methylphenidate HCl	Ritalin	CNS stimulant
methylprednisolone	Medrol	Corticosteroid
metroprolol	Lopressor	Cardiac drug
metroprolol succinate	Toprol-XL	Cardiac drug
mometasone furoate	Elocon	Anti-inflammatory agent
mupirocin	Bactroban	Antibiotic
nabumetone	Relafen	Nonsteroidal anti-inflammatory agent
naproxen	Naprosyn	Nonsteroidal anti-inflammatory agent
nefazodone HCl	Serzone	Antidepressant
neomycin	Neosporin	Antibiotic
nifedipine	Adalat, Procardia	Cardiac drug
nitrofurantoin	Macrobid	Antibiotic
nitroglycerin	Nitro-Dur, Nitrostat	Vasodilating agent
nizatidine	Axid	GI drug (H_2 antagonist)

Generic Name	Brand Name	Type of Drug
ofloxacin	Floxin	Antibiotic
omeprazole	Prilosec	GI drug (H_2 antagonist)
orphenadrine citrate	Norflex	Skeletal muscle relaxant
oxaprozin	Daypro	Nonsteroid anti-inflammatory agent
oxycodone & APAP	Percocert	Opiate agonist, analgesic
oxycodone HCl & APAP	Roxicet	Opiate agonist, analgesic
oxycodone with ASA	Percodan	Opiate agonist, analgesic
paroxetine HCl	Paxil	Antidepressant
penicillin v potassium	Veetids	Antibiotic
pentoxifylline	Trental	Hemorheologic agent
phentermine HCl	Fastin	Anorexiant
phenytoin	Dilantin	Anticonvulsant
potassium chloride	K-LOA, Klor-Con, Klorvess, Micro-K, K-Dur, K-Lor, K-Lyte/CL, K-Tab	Potassium supplement
pravastatine sodium	Pravachol	Lipid lowering drug
prednisone	Deltasone, Meticorten, Orasone	Corticosteroid
promethazine HCl	Phenergan	Antihistamine/antiemetic
propoxyphene napsylate	Darvocet-N	Opiate agonist, analgesic
quinapril HCl	Accupril	Cardiac drug

Generic Name	Brand Name	Type of Drug
ramipril	Altace	Cardiac drug
ranitidine	Zantac	GI drug (H_2 antagonist)
resperidone	Risperdal	Antipsycotic drug
robitussin, humibid	Guaifenesin	Expectorant
salmeterol	Serevent	Bronchodilator
sertraline HCl	Zoloft	Antidepressant
simvastatine	Zocor	Lipid lowering drug
sumatriptan succinate	Imitrex	Migraine analgesic
tamoxifen citrate	Nolvadex	Antineoplastic hormone
temazepam	Restoril	Sedative/hypnotic (benzodiazepine)
terazosin	Hytrin	Antihypertensive
terbinafine HCl	Lamisil	Antifungal
ticlopidine HCl	Ticlid	Platelet aggregation inhibitor
timolol muleate	Timoptic-XE	Antiglaucoma
tobramycin & dexamethasone	Tobradex	Anti-inflammatory/antibiotic
tramadol HCl	Ultram	Opiate agonist, analgesic
trazodone HCl	Desyrel	Antidepressant
triamcinolone acetonide	Azmacort	Corticosteroid
triamterene & HCTZ	Dyazide	Diuretic
triamterent & HCTZ	Maxzide	Diuretic
trimethoprim & sulfa	Bactrim	Antibiotic

Generic Name	Brand Name	Type of Drug
venlafaxine	Effexor	Antidepressant
verapamil HCl	Calan, Isoptin	Cardiac drug
warfarin sodium	Coumadin	Anticoagulant
zolpiden tartrate	Ambien	Sedative/hypnotic

Common Charting Abbreviations

Common Charting Abbreviations

$\bar{a}$	Before
AAA	Abdominal aortic aneurysm
abd	Abdominal
ABG's	Arterial blood gases
ac	Before meals
a.d.	Right ear
ad lib	As desired
AMA	Against medical advice
A.P.	Apical pulse
a.s.	Left ear
ASAP	As soon as possible
a.u.	Both ears
ax	Axillary
bid	Twice a day
bilat	Bilateral
BP	Blood pressure
BS	Bowel sounds
BSP	Bowel sounds present
$\bar{c}$	With
Ca	Cancer
cap	Capsule
CC	Chief complaint
cl	Clear
CNS	Central nervous system

c/o	Complains of
C-Spine	Cervical
CVA	Cerebral vascular accident
DC	Discontinue; discharge
diff	Difficulty
D.M.	Diabetes mellitus
DOA	Dead on arrival
DOE	Dyspnea on exertion
dsg	Dressing
DT's	Delirium tremens
Dx	Diagnosis
EBL	Estimated blood loss
ECG, EKG	Electrocardiogram
EEG	Electroencephalogram
E&R	Equal and reactive
est	Estimated
ETA	Estimated time of arrival
ETOH	Ethyl alcohol
F.B.	Foreign body
FHT's	Fetal heart tones
Fld's	Fluids
FUO	Fever of unknown origin
FX	Fracture
G	Gravida
GB	Gallbladder
gcs	Glasgow coma scale

GI	Gastrointestinal
GSW	Gunshot wound
gtt(s)	Drop(s)
GU	Genitourinary
h	Hour
h/a	Headache
Hct	Hematocrit
Hgb	Hemoglobin
Hosp	Hospital
HTN	Hypertension
HS	At bedtime
Hx	History
IC	Intracardiac
ID	Intradermal
IM	Intramuscular
IV	Intravenous
IVP	IV push
IVPB	IV piggyback
jt	Joint
l	Liter
L	Left
lac	Laceration
lg	Large
liq	Liquid
LLE	Left lower extremity
LLQ	Left lower quadrant

LMP	Last menstrual period
LOC	Loss of consciousness, level of consciousness
L-Spine	Lumbar
LUE	Left upper extremity
LUQ	Left upper quadrant
med(s)	Medication(s)
menst	Menstrual
mod	Moderate
mult	Multiple
NAD	No acute distress
nb	Newborn
NC	Nasal cannula
neg	Negative
N/G	Nasogastric
NIAL	Not in active labor
noc	Night
NPO	Nothing by mouth
NROM	Normal range of motion
NS	Normal saline
NSVD	Normal spontaneous vaginal delivery
N&T	Numbness and tingling
N&V	Nausea and vomiting
O	None
occ	Occasional

OD	Overdose
o.d.	Right eye
o.s.	Left eye
o.u.	Each eye
P	Pulse
$\bar{p}$	After
PB	Piggyback
p.c.	After meals
PE	Pulmonary edema, pulmonary embolism
ped	Pedestrian
PEEP	Positive end expiratory pressure
PERL(A)	Pupils equal, reactive to light (with accommodation)
PEARL	Pupils equal and reactive to light
PND	Paroxysmal nocturnal dyspnea
po	By mouth
poss	Possible
POV	Privately owned vehicle
PP	Postpartum
PR	Per rectum
prn	When necessary, as needed
prox	Proximal
pt	Patient
PTA	Prior to arrival (admission)

q	Each, every
qid	Four times a day
qod	Every other day
R	Right; rectal; respiration
RBC's	Red blood cells
RDS	Respiratory disease syndrome
re	Regarding
req	Request
RLE	Right lower extremity
RLQ	Right lower quadrant
R/O	Rule out
ROJM	Range of joint motion
ROM	Range of motion
RUE	Right upper extremity
RUQ	Right upper quadrant
Rx	Treatment
SAH	Subarachnoid hemorrhage
SBO	Small bowel obstruction
SL	Sublingual
sl	Slight
sm	Small
SOB	Short of breath
sol	Solution
SQ	Subcutaneous
$\bar{s}$	Without
S-Spine	Sacral

ss	Half
STAT	Immediately
STD	Sexually transmitted disease
Supp	Suppository
SW	Stab wound
Sx/Sx	Signs and symptoms
T	Temperature
Tab	Tablet
TB	Tuberculosis
TIA	Transient ischemic attack
tid	Three times a day
TPR	Temperature, pulse, respiration
tr	Tincture
T-Spine	Thoracic
U/A	Urinalysis
u.d.	As directed
UGI	Upper gastrointestinal
Unc	Unconscious
URI	Upper respiratory infection
URP	Unreliable patient
UTI	Urinary tract infection
VD	Venereal disease
WB	Whole blood
WBC's	White blood cells
W/C	Wheelchair

WD/WN	Well developed/well nourished
WNL	Within normal limits
wt	Weight
y/o	Years old

Bibliography

Bibliography

Akron General Medical Center: <u>Formulary of Drugs 1996/1997 Handbook,</u> Lexi-Comp Inc. Hudson, Ohio, 1996.

American College of Emergency Physicians, Pons P.T., Cason D., Editors: <u>Paramedic Field Care: A Complaint-Based Approach,</u> American College of Emergency Physicians, 1997.

American College of Surgeons, Committee on Trauma: <u>Advanced Trauma Life Support for Doctors Student Course Manual,</u> American College of Surgeons, 1997.

American Heart Association: <u>Advanced Cardiac Life Support,</u> American Heart Association, Dallas, 1997.

American Heart Association and American Academy of Pediatrics: <u>Textbook of Pediatric Advanced Life Support,</u> American Heart Association, Dallas, 1994.

Butman A.M., Martin S.W., et al: <u>Comprehensive Guide to Pre-Hospital Skills: A Skills Manual for EMT-Basic, EMT-Intermediate, EMT-Paramedic,</u> Emergency Training, Akron, Ohio, 1995.

Caroline N.L.: <u>Emergency Care in the Streets,</u> 5th Edition, Little Brown, 1995.

DiGregorio G.J., Barbieri E.J.: <u>Handbook of Commonly Prescribed Drugs,</u> 9th Edition, Medical Surveillance, Inc., West Chester, PA, 1994.

Dubin D.: <u>Rapid Interpretation of EKG's,</u> 5th Edition, Cover Publishing Company, Tampa, FL, 1996.

Hoppenfeld S.: <u>Physical Examination of the Spine and Extremitie</u>s, Appleton-Century-Crofts, Prentice Hall, Inc., 1976.

Keen J.H., et al: Mosby's Critical Care and Emergency Drug Reference, Mosby, Inc., St. Louis, 1994.

Medical Economics Company: Physician's Desk Reference, 52nd Edition, Medical Economics Company, Montvale, NJ, 1998.

Phalen T.: The 12 Lead ECG in Acute Myocardial Infaction, Mosby, Inc., St. Louis,1996.

Rasch P.J., Burke R.K.: Kinesiology and Applied Anatomy, 7th Edition, Lea and Febiger, Philadelphia, PA, 1989.

Stutz D.R., et al: Hazardous Materials Injuries: A Handbook for Pre-Hospital Care, Bradford Communications Corporation, Greenbelt, MD, 1982.

Takolomo, C.K., Hodding J.H., Kraus, D.M.: Pediatric Dosage Handbook, 4th Edition, Lexi-Comp, Inc., Hudson, OH, 1997.

Tintinalli J.E., et al: American College of Emergency Physicians, Emergency Medicine: A Comprehensive Study Guide, 3rd Edition, McGraw-Hill, 1992.

UDL Laboratories Inc.: Generic-Brand Comparison Handbook, UDL Laboratories, Inc., Loves Park, IL, 1997.

United States Department of Transportation (USDOT): Emergency Response Guidebook, 1993.

SKIDMORE-ROTH PUBLISHING INC.

400 Inverness Drive South, Suite 260
Englewood, CO 80112
Ph. 1-800-825-3150

QTY	TITLE	PRICE	TOTAL
	Pediatric Nursing Care Plans, (2nd ed.), Jaffe 1998	$38.95	
	Pediatric Nurse's Survival Guide, Rebeschi 1996	$29.95	
	Body in Brief (3rd ed.), Rayman 1997	$35.95	
	Diagnostic and Lab Cards, (3rd ed.), Skidmore-Roth 1998	$29.95	
	Drug Comparison Handbook, (3rd ed.), Reilly 1998	$36.95	
	Obstetric Nursing Outline, (2nd ed.), Masten 1997	$23.95	
	Pediatric Nursing Outline, (2nd ed.), Froese-Fretz et al 1998	$23.95	
	Critical Care Nursing Care Plans, Comer 1998	$38.95	
	RN-NCLEX Review Cards (3rd ed.), Goodner 1998	$32.95	
Colorado residents add sales tax. Shipping & handling will be added. Prices subject to change without notice. (continued on next page)		Subtotal	
		Tax	
		S&H	
		Total	

Name		
Company		
Address		
City		State
Zip		Phone
Check enclosed	Visa	Master Card
Credit Card Number		
Cardholder Name		
Signature		Exp.

For faster service call 1-800-825-3150. Orders are accepted by mail with payment.
Skidmore-Roth Publishing, Inc.
400 Inverness Drive South, Suite 260
Englewood, CO 80112

Visit our website at:
http://www.skidmore-roth.com